THE ENERVATE EFFECT RECHARGING YOUR LIFE'S BATTERY

DIPAN KUMAR DAS

SUDIP KUMAR DAS

To all those who have ever felt drained, overwhelmed, or depleted, this book is dedicated to you. May its pages serve as a beacon of hope and inspiration, guiding you toward a life filled with renewed energy, vitality, and joy. You are deserving of the love, care, and attention you give to others, and may you always remember to prioritize your own well-being along your journey. This book is for you.

Foreword

In the hustle and bustle of today's world, it's all too easy to find ourselves running on empty, constantly striving to meet the demands of work, family, and daily life. In the midst of this chaos, the importance of self-care and energy renewal often takes a backseat.

In "The Enervate Effect: Recharging Your Life's Battery," offers a timely and insightful exploration into the transformative power of prioritizing our own well-being. Through a blend of personal anecdotes, scientific research, and practical advice, invites readers on a journey of self-discovery and renewal.

Drawing upon years of experience in the fields of psychology, wellness, and personal development, provides readers with a roadmap for reclaiming their energy and vitality. From the importance of rest and relaxation to the role of nutrition and exercise in maintaining optimal health, this book offers a comprehensive guide to living a life filled with purpose, passion, and joy.

As you embark on this journey of exploration, I encourage you to approach these pages with an open mind and a willingness to embrace change. May you find inspiration, guidance, and empowerment within these words, and may you emerge from this journey with a renewed sense of energy and purpose.

Preface

Welcome to "The Enervate Effect: Recharging Your Life's Battery." As you hold this book in your hands, you're embarking on a journey toward greater energy, vitality, and well-being.

In today's fast-paced world, it's all too easy to feel drained and depleted, constantly juggling the demands of work, family, and personal life. But what if I told you that it doesn't have to be this way? What if I told you that you have the power to reclaim your energy and live a life filled with passion and purpose?

In the pages that follow, I'll share with you the insights, strategies, and practices that have helped me and countless others break free from the cycle of exhaustion and embrace a life of vitality. Drawing upon the latest research in psychology, neuroscience, and wellness, I'll guide you step-by-step through the process of identifying the sources of energy drain in your life and implementing practical solutions for recharging your batteries.

But this book isn't just about quick fixes and temporary solutions. It's about cultivating habits and practices that will sustain you for a lifetime. It's about reclaiming your power and prioritizing your own well-being. And most importantly, it's about recognizing that you are worthy of the love, care, and attention you give to others.

As you read through these pages, I encourage you to approach this journey with an open mind and a willingness to embrace change. You may encounter challenges along the way, but know that you are not alone. I'll be here to guide you every step of the way.

So let's embark on this journey together. Let's reclaim our energy, reignite our passion, and live our lives to the fullest. The power to transform your life is within your grasp. Are you ready to seize it?

Prologue

In the chaos of modern life, it's all too easy to lose sight of ourselves amidst the demands and distractions that surround us. We find ourselves caught in a relentless cycle of busyness, constantly striving to keep up with the never-ending to-do lists and responsibilities that seem to consume our days.

But amid the chaos, there is a quiet voice within us—a voice that whispers of a different way of living. It speaks of a life filled with energy, vitality, and purpose. A life where we prioritize our own well-being and nourish our souls with the care and attention they deserve.

"The Enervate Effect: Recharging Your Life's Battery" is a testament to the power of that quiet voice. It is a call to action—a reminder that we hold within us the power to transform our lives from the inside out.

In the pages that follow, we'll embark on a journey of self-discovery and renewal. We'll explore the sources of energy drain in our lives and uncover practical strategies for recharging our batteries and reclaiming our vitality.

But more than that, we'll delve into the deeper truths of what it means to live a life of meaning and purpose. We'll explore the connections between our physical, mental, and spiritual well-being and discover how nurturing each of these aspects of ourselves can lead to a life of fulfillment and joy.

So join me as we embark on this journey together. Let us cast aside the shackles of exhaustion and embrace a life filled with energy, passion, and purpose. The journey may be challenging at times, but know that you are not alone. Together, we will navigate the twists and turns of this path, emerging stronger, wiser, and more vibrant than ever before.

Overcoming Obstacles And Staying On Track

8.

The Enervate Effect In Action

Epilogue

CHAPTER ONE

Understanding Energy Drain

Recognizing the Signs of Enervation

Enervation, or the state of being drained of energy or vitality, can manifest in various ways, both physically and mentally. Here are some common signs to look out for:

Fatigue: Feeling constantly tired or lacking energy, even after getting enough sleep or rest.

Difficulty Concentrating: Struggling to focus or concentrate on tasks, experiencing brain fog, or having trouble making decisions.

Irritability: Being easily annoyed, agitated, or short-tempered, often over minor issues.

Muscle Weakness: Feeling physically weak or experiencing muscle fatigue even with minimal exertion.

Decreased Motivation: Losing interest in activities you once enjoyed, feeling demotivated or apathetic towards goals or responsibilities.

Poor Sleep: Having trouble falling asleep, staying asleep, or experiencing restless sleep patterns.

Increased Sensitivity to Stress: Finding it difficult to cope with stressors, feeling overwhelmed by everyday tasks, or experiencing heightened anxiety.

Physical Symptoms: Experiencing headaches, body aches, or gastrointestinal issues without any apparent cause.

Decreased Immunity: Getting sick frequently or taking longer to recover from illnesses.

Social Withdrawal: Withdrawing from social interactions, preferring to isolate oneself rather than engage with others.

Changes in Appetite: Eating significantly more or less than usual, or experiencing changes in cravings.

Emotional Instability: Feeling more emotional than usual, experiencing mood swings, or feeling on edge without a clear reason.

If you notice several of these signs persisting over a prolonged period, it may be a good idea to seek support from a healthcare professional. Enervation can have various underlying causes, including physical health issues, psychological factors, lifestyle habits, or a combination of these factors. Addressing the root cause is essential for regaining energy and vitality.

Exploring the Impact of Stress and Overexertion

Stress and overexertion can have significant impacts on both physical and mental well-being. Here's an exploration of their effects:

Physical Impact:

Weakened Immune System: Prolonged stress can suppress the immune system, making individuals more susceptible to illnesses and infections.

Musculoskeletal Issues: Overexertion can lead to muscle strains, sprains, or even more severe injuries like tendonitis or stress fractures.

Cardiovascular Problems: Chronic stress can contribute to high blood pressure, heart disease, and increased risk of heart attacks or strokes.

Gastrointestinal Distress: Stress can exacerbate digestive issues such as irritable bowel syndrome (IBS), acid reflux, or ulcers.

Sleep Disorders: Both stress and overexertion can disrupt sleep patterns, leading to insomnia or poor-quality sleep, which in turn can further exacerbate stress levels.

Mental Impact:

Anxiety and Depression: Chronic stress can contribute to the development or worsening of anxiety and depression disorders.

Cognitive Functioning: Stress can impair memory, concentration, and decision-making abilities, affecting overall cognitive performance.

Mood Changes: Overexertion and stress can lead to irritability, mood swings, and feelings of frustration or hopelessness.

Burnout: Overexertion, especially when combined with chronic stress, can lead to burnout—a state of physical, emotional, and mental exhaustion often accompanied by feelings of detachment and reduced performance.

Social Withdrawal: Stress and overexertion can diminish the desire or ability to engage in social activities, leading to isolation and loneliness.

Behavioral Impact:

Decreased Productivity: Overexertion and stress can impair performance at work or school, leading to decreased productivity and efficiency.

Substance Abuse: Some individuals may turn to alcohol, drugs, or other substances as a way to cope with stress or mask its effects, which can lead to addiction issues.

Poor Coping Mechanisms: Stressful situations may lead to unhealthy coping mechanisms such as overeating, undereating, or engaging in risky behaviors.

Relationship Strain: Stress and overexertion can put a strain on personal relationships, leading to conflicts, misunderstandings, or withdrawal from loved ones.

Cognitive Impact:

Impaired Decision-Making: Stress can cloud judgment and impair decision-making abilities, leading to poor choices or indecision.

Difficulty Concentrating: Overexertion and stress can make it challenging to focus on tasks or absorb new information, affecting learning and performance.

Emotional Impact:

Heightened Emotional Sensitivity: Stress and overexertion can make individuals more emotionally reactive, leading to heightened sensitivity to criticism or perceived slights.

Feelings of Overwhelm: When stress and overexertion become overwhelming, individuals may feel a sense of helplessness or hopelessness about their circumstances.

Loss of Enjoyment: Engaging in activities that were once enjoyable may feel like a burden or obligation when under significant stress or overexertion.

Long-Term Impact:

Chronic Health Conditions: Prolonged exposure to stress and overexertion is associated with an increased risk of developing chronic health conditions such as obesity, diabetes, and autoimmune disorders.

Accelerated Aging: Chronic stress can accelerate the aging process at a cellular level, leading to premature aging and increased vulnerability to age-related diseases.

Decreased Quality of Life: Persistent stress and overexertion can erode overall quality of life, diminishing enjoyment of daily activities and impairing overall well-being.

Interpersonal Impact:

Communication Issues: Stress and overexertion can hinder effective communication, leading to misunderstandings or conflicts in personal and professional relationships.

Lack of Support: When individuals are overwhelmed by stress or overexertion, they may withdraw from social support networks, further exacerbating feelings of isolation and loneliness.

Financial Impact:

Work Performance: Stress and overexertion can impact job performance, potentially leading to missed deadlines, decreased productivity, or even job loss.

Healthcare Costs: Chronic stress-related health conditions can result in increased healthcare expenses due to frequent doctor visits, medications, and treatments.

It's essential to recognize the signs of stress and overexertion early on and take proactive steps to manage them. This might include practicing relaxation techniques, setting boundaries, prioritizing self-care, seeking support from friends or professionals, and making adjustments to lifestyle and workload as needed.

Identifying Sources of Energy Drain in Everyday Life

Identifying sources of energy drain in everyday life is crucial for maintaining overall well-being and productivity. Here are some common culprits:

Physical Factors:

Poor Sleep Habits: Inadequate sleep or irregular sleep patterns can leave you feeling tired and drained throughout the day.

Unhealthy Diet: Consuming excessive amounts of processed foods, sugar, caffeine, or alcohol can negatively impact energy levels.

Lack of Exercise: Sedentary lifestyles can contribute to feelings of lethargy and low energy. Regular physical activity is essential for boosting energy levels.

Dehydration: Not drinking enough water can lead to fatigue and decreased cognitive function.

Psychological Factors:

Stress: Chronic stress from work, relationships, or financial worries can drain mental and emotional energy.

Perfectionism: Setting unrealistic expectations for yourself can lead to constant stress and burnout.

Overwhelm: Trying to juggle too many responsibilities at once can leave you feeling mentally exhausted.

Negative Thinking: Dwelling on negative thoughts or emotions can drain mental energy and reduce motivation.

Lack of Purpose: Feeling unfulfilled or lacking direction in life can contribute to a sense of lethargy and apathy.

Environmental Factors:

Clutter: A cluttered or disorganized environment can create mental chaos and drain your energy.

Toxic Relationships: Spending time with negative or unsupportive people can leave you feeling drained and emotionally exhausted.

Noise Pollution: Excessive noise or distractions in your environment can make it difficult to concentrate and drain your mental energy.

Poor Lighting: Insufficient natural light or harsh artificial lighting can affect mood and energy levels.

Lifestyle Habits:

Overcommitting: Saying yes to too many obligations or activities can spread you thin and deplete your energy.

Procrastination: Putting off tasks until the last minute can create unnecessary stress and drain mental energy.

Technology Overuse: Spending excessive time on screens, especially before bed, can disrupt sleep patterns and drain mental energy.

Neglecting Self-Care: Failing to prioritize self-care activities such as relaxation, hobbies, and socializing can lead to burnout and decreased energy levels.

Health Issues:

Chronic Illness: Underlying health conditions such as thyroid disorders, anemia, or chronic fatigue syndrome can cause persistent fatigue and low energy.

Mental Health Disorders: Conditions like depression, anxiety, or bipolar disorder can significantly impact energy levels and overall functioning.

By identifying these sources of energy drain, you can take proactive steps to address them and cultivate habits that promote sustained energy and well-being. This might include prioritizing sleep, adopting a balanced diet, managing stress effectively, setting boundaries, and seeking support when needed.

Here are specific examples of sources of energy drain in various aspects of life:

Physical Factors:

Poor Sleep Habits: Staying up late watching TV or scrolling through your phone, leading to insufficient sleep and feeling groggy the next day.

Unhealthy Eating: Consuming a diet high in processed foods, sugar, and caffeine, resulting in energy crashes and mood swings.

Lack of Exercise: Sitting at a desk all day without incorporating movement breaks or regular exercise, leading to muscle stiffness and decreased energy levels.

Dehydration: Not drinking enough water throughout the day, resulting in feelings of fatigue and difficulty concentrating.

Psychological Factors:

Workplace Stress: Constantly worrying about meeting deadlines, dealing with demanding clients, or navigating office politics, leading to mental exhaustion.

Perfectionism: Spending excessive time and energy striving for perfection in tasks or projects, resulting in burnout and diminished motivation.

Overwhelm: Feeling overwhelmed by a never-ending to-do list or multiple competing priorities, making it difficult to focus and draining mental energy.

Rumination: Obsessively dwelling on past mistakes or worrying about future outcomes, leading to increased anxiety and depleted mental reserves.

Environmental Factors:

Cluttered Workspace: Working in a cluttered or disorganized environment, causing distractions and making it challenging to stay focused.

Toxic Relationships: Interacting with negative or unsupportive individuals who drain your energy with their constant complaints or drama.

Noisy Environment: Working or living in a noisy area with constant background noise, making it difficult to concentrate and draining mental energy.

Poor Lighting: Working in a dimly lit room or spending too much time under harsh fluorescent lights, leading to eye strain and fatigue.

Lifestyle Habits:

Overcommitting: Saying yes to every social invitation, volunteer opportunity, or work project, resulting in feeling overwhelmed and spread too thin.

Procrastination: Putting off important tasks until the last minute, causing stress and anxiety as deadlines approach, and draining mental energy.

Screen Time: Spending hours mindlessly scrolling through social media or binge-watching TV shows, leading to disrupted sleep patterns and decreased energy levels.

Neglecting Self-Care: Failing to prioritize activities that recharge and rejuvenate you, such as exercise, hobbies, or spending time with loved ones, resulting in feeling depleted and burnt out.

These examples illustrate how various aspects of life can contribute to energy drain, highlighting the importance of recognizing these factors and implementing strategies to mitigate their impact on overall well-being.

CHAPTER TWO

The Power of Rest and Recovery

Embracing the Importance of Restorative Practices

Embracing restorative practices is crucial for maintaining balance, replenishing energy, and promoting overall well-being. Here's why they're important:

Physical Health:

Improved Sleep Quality: Restorative practices such as establishing a consistent bedtime routine and incorporating relaxation techniques can enhance sleep quality, leading to better physical health and energy levels.

Reduced Risk of Burnout: Taking breaks, practicing mindfulness, and engaging in restorative activities can prevent burnout by allowing the body to recharge and recover from stress and exertion.

Mental Health:

Stress Reduction: Restorative practices like meditation, deep breathing exercises, and spending time in nature can reduce stress levels, promote relaxation, and improve mental clarity.

Enhanced Resilience: Engaging in activities that foster a sense of calm and well-being can enhance resilience and equip individuals with coping mechanisms to better navigate challenges and setbacks.

Emotional Well-being:

Increased Emotional Awareness: Restorative practices such as journaling or therapy can help individuals process emotions, cultivate self-awareness, and develop healthier coping strategies.

Promotion of Positive Emotions: Activities like spending time with loved ones, practicing gratitude, or pursuing hobbies can boost mood and foster feelings of joy and fulfillment.

Cognitive Function:

Enhanced Focus and Concentration: Taking regular breaks and engaging in restorative activities can improve focus, concentration, and cognitive function, leading to increased productivity and efficiency.

Stimulation of Creativity: Restorative practices that encourage relaxation and free-flowing thought, such as mindfulness or artistic pursuits, can stimulate creativity and innovation.

Social Connection:

Fostering Relationships: Spending quality time with friends and family, engaging in meaningful conversations, and participating in community activities are restorative practices that nurture social connections and support networks.

Reducing Feelings of Isolation: Restorative activities that involve social interaction can alleviate feelings of loneliness and strengthen a sense of belonging and connection.

Overall Well-being:

Enhanced Quality of Life: Prioritizing restorative practices contributes to overall well-being by promoting physical health, mental clarity, emotional resilience, and social connection.

Prevention of Chronic Health Conditions: Chronic stress and overexertion are linked to various health issues. Embracing restorative practices can reduce the risk of developing chronic health conditions and improve long-term health outcomes.

By embracing restorative practices, individuals can cultivate a healthier, more balanced lifestyle, enabling them to thrive personally and professionally while effectively managing the demands of everyday life.

Strategies for Quality Sleep and Rejuvenation

Quality sleep and rejuvenation are essential for overall health and well-being. Here are some strategies to promote restful sleep and rejuvenation:

Establish a Sleep Routine:

Consistent Bedtime: Go to bed and wake up at the same time every day, even on weekends, to regulate your body's internal clock.

Bedtime Ritual: Develop a relaxing pre-sleep routine, such as taking a warm bath, reading a book, or practicing relaxation exercises, to signal to your body that it's time to wind down.

Limit Screen Time: Avoid electronic devices such as smartphones, tablets, and computers at least an hour before bedtime, as the blue light emitted can disrupt sleep patterns.

Create a Restful Sleep Environment:

Comfortable Bedding: Invest in a comfortable mattress, pillows, and bedding that support restful sleep and promote proper alignment of the spine.

Dark and Quiet: Make your bedroom conducive to sleep by minimizing noise and light. Consider using blackout curtains, white noise machines, or earplugs to create a peaceful environment.

Optimal Temperature: Keep your bedroom cool and comfortable, ideally between 60-67 degrees Fahrenheit (15-19 degrees Celsius), to promote restful sleep.

Practice Healthy Sleep Habits:

Limit Caffeine and Alcohol: Avoid consuming caffeine and alcohol close to bedtime, as they can disrupt sleep patterns and reduce sleep quality.

Regular Exercise: Engage in regular physical activity during the day, but avoid vigorous exercise close to bedtime, as it can interfere with sleep.

Watch Your Diet: Avoid heavy meals, spicy foods, and excessive fluid intake before bedtime to prevent discomfort and nighttime awakenings.

Manage Stress and Relaxation:

Stress Management: Practice stress-reduction techniques such as mindfulness meditation, deep breathing exercises, or progressive muscle relaxation to calm the mind and promote relaxation before bedtime.

Journaling: Spend a few minutes journaling before bed to unload any thoughts or worries on paper, helping to clear your mind and promote relaxation.

Yoga or Stretching: Incorporate gentle stretching or yoga poses into your bedtime routine to release tension from the body and prepare for sleep.

Seek Professional Help if Needed:

Consult a Healthcare Professional: If you consistently struggle with sleep issues despite trying various strategies, consult a healthcare professional to rule out any underlying sleep disorders or medical conditions.

Therapy or Counseling: Consider seeking therapy or counseling if stress, anxiety, or other emotional issues are interfering with your ability to sleep well.

By incorporating these strategies into your daily routine, you can create an environment conducive to quality sleep and rejuvenation, promoting overall health and well-being.

Techniques for Relaxation and Stress Reduction

Here are some techniques for relaxation and stress reduction:

Mindfulness and Meditation:

Deep Breathing: Practice deep breathing exercises, such as diaphragmatic breathing or box breathing, to activate the body's relaxation response and reduce stress.

Body Scan Meditation: Engage in a body scan meditation, where you systematically focus on each part of your body, releasing tension and promoting relaxation.

Mindful Awareness: Practice mindfulness by bringing your attention to the present moment without judgment, observing thoughts, emotions, and sensations as they arise.

Progressive Muscle Relaxation (PMR):

Muscle Tension and Release: Systematically tense and then relax different muscle groups in your body, starting from your toes and working your way up to your head, to release physical tension and induce relaxation.

Focused Relaxation: Direct your attention to areas of the body where you feel tension or discomfort, consciously releasing tension and allowing those muscles to relax.

Visualization and Imagery:

Guided Imagery: Listen to or create guided imagery scripts that transport you to peaceful and calming settings, such as a beach or forest, allowing your mind to relax and unwind.

Positive Visualization: Visualize yourself in a calm and relaxing environment or engaging in activities that bring you joy and peace, allowing your mind to focus on positive thoughts and emotions.

Relaxation Techniques:

Progressive Relaxation: Engage in activities that promote relaxation and well-being, such as taking a warm bath, listening to soothing music, or practicing gentle yoga.

Aromatherapy: Use essential oils such as lavender, chamomile, or bergamot, which are known for their calming and stress-relieving properties, either through diffusion, inhalation, or topical application.

Mindful Movement:

Yoga: Practice gentle yoga sequences or restorative yoga poses that focus on deep breathing, stretching, and relaxation, helping to release physical tension and promote mental calmness.

Tai Chi or Qigong: Engage in slow, flowing movements and deep breathing exercises that promote relaxation, balance, and mindfulness.

Lifestyle Habits:

Prioritize Self-Care: Make time for activities that bring you joy and relaxation, such as spending time in nature, pursuing hobbies, or connecting with loved ones.

Set Boundaries: Learn to say no to excessive commitments and prioritize tasks that are essential, allowing you to manage stress and prevent overwhelm.

Professional Support:

Therapy or Counseling: Consider seeking support from a therapist or counselor who can provide strategies for coping with stress, managing emotions, and promoting relaxation.

Mindfulness-Based Stress Reduction (MBSR): Participate in MBSR programs or workshops, which combine mindfulness meditation, yoga, and education to help individuals manage stress and improve well-being.

By incorporating these techniques into your daily routine, you can cultivate a greater sense of relaxation, reduce stress levels, and promote overall well-being.

Here are some of the best tips for relaxation and stress reduction:

1. Practice Deep Breathing:

Technique: Take slow, deep breaths, focusing on fully inhaling and exhaling. Try the 4-7-8 technique: Inhale for 4 seconds, hold for 7 seconds, and exhale for 8 seconds.

Why It Works: Deep breathing activates the body's relaxation response, calming the nervous system and reducing stress.

2. Mindfulness Meditation:

Practice: Set aside a few minutes each day to sit quietly and focus on your breath or a specific sensation. Notice when your mind wanders and gently bring your attention back to the present moment.

Why It Works: Mindfulness meditation helps cultivate awareness and acceptance of the present moment, reducing anxiety and promoting relaxation.

3. Progressive Muscle Relaxation (PMR):

Technique: Tense and then relax different muscle groups in your body, starting from your toes and working your way up to your head. Hold the tension for a few seconds before releasing.

Why It Works: PMR helps release physical tension and promotes deep relaxation throughout the body.

4. Engage in Physical Activity:

Activity: Take a walk, go for a run, or engage in any form of exercise you enjoy. Even a short burst of physical activity can help reduce stress and improve mood.

Why It Works: Exercise releases endorphins, chemicals in the brain that act as natural painkillers and mood elevators, promoting relaxation and well-being.

5. Practice Gratitude:

Activity: Take a few moments each day to reflect on things you're grateful for. Write them down in a journal or simply think about them silently.

Why It Works: Gratitude practice shifts your focus from negative to positive emotions, reducing stress and increasing feelings of contentment and happiness.

6. Spend Time in Nature:

Activity: Take a walk in the park, go for a hike, or simply sit outside and enjoy the natural surroundings.

Why It Works: Spending time in nature has been shown to lower cortisol levels (the stress hormone) and promote feelings of relaxation and well-being.

7. Limit Screen Time:

Practice: Set boundaries around your screen time, especially before bed. Create a digital curfew and engage in calming activities instead, such as reading or listening to soothing music.

Why It Works: Excessive screen time, particularly before bed, can disrupt sleep patterns and increase stress levels. Limiting screen time promotes relaxation and better sleep quality.

8. Connect with Others:

Activity: Spend time with friends, family, or loved ones. Engage in meaningful conversations, share laughter, or simply enjoy each other's company.

Why It Works: Social connections are essential for emotional well-being. Spending time with others can provide support, reduce feelings of loneliness, and promote relaxation.

9. Set Realistic Goals:

Practice: Break larger tasks into smaller, manageable goals. Prioritize tasks based on importance and urgency, and be realistic about what you can accomplish in a given time frame.

Why It Works: Setting realistic goals reduces feelings of overwhelm and helps you stay focused and motivated, ultimately reducing stress.

10. Prioritize Self-Care:

Activity: Make time for activities that nourish your mind, body, and soul. Whether it's taking a bubble bath, reading a book, or indulging in a hobby, prioritize self-care regularly.

Why It Works: Self-care activities replenish your energy, reduce stress levels, and promote overall well-being.

11. Practice Time Management:

Strategy: Break your day into manageable chunks, schedule regular breaks, and prioritize tasks. Use time-blocking techniques to allocate specific time slots for different activities.

Why It Works: Effective time management reduces feelings of overwhelm and helps you feel more in control, ultimately reducing stress.

12. Listen to Music:

Activity: Create a playlist of calming or uplifting music and listen to it when you're feeling stressed or overwhelmed. Pay attention to how different types of music affect your mood.

Why It Works: Music has a powerful effect on emotions and can help reduce stress, promote relaxation, and improve mood.

13. Practice Self-Compassion:

Activity: Treat yourself with kindness and understanding, especially when facing difficult situations or setbacks. Practice self-compassionate self-talk and avoid harsh self-criticism.

Why It Works: Self-compassion fosters resilience, reduces negative emotions, and promotes a sense of well-being, even in challenging circumstances.

14. Laugh Often:

Activity: Watch a funny movie or TV show, spend time with friends who make you laugh, or seek out humorous content online.

Why It Works: Laughter triggers the release of endorphins, promoting relaxation and reducing stress. It also helps shift perspective and provides a temporary escape from stressors.

15. Engage in Creative Activities:

Activity: Paint, draw, write, cook, or engage in any other creative activity you enjoy. Focus on the process rather than the outcome.

Why It Works: Creative activities provide an outlet for self-expression, reduce stress, and promote relaxation by engaging the mind in a fulfilling and enjoyable task.

16. Practice Mindful Eating:

Activity: Slow down and savor each bite during meals. Pay attention to the taste, texture, and aroma of your food, and listen to your body's hunger and fullness cues.

Why It Works: Mindful eating promotes relaxation, reduces stress-related eating, and fosters a healthier relationship with food and body.

17. Spend Time with Pets:

Activity: If you have a pet, spend quality time with them engaging in activities such as playing, cuddling, or going for a walk together.

Why It Works: Interacting with pets has been shown to reduce stress levels, lower blood pressure, and increase feelings of happiness and relaxation.

18. Practice Gratitude Journaling:

Activity: Keep a gratitude journal and write down three things you're grateful for each day. Focus on specific details and reflect on why you're thankful for each item.

Why It Works: Gratitude journaling shifts your focus from negativity to positivity, promotes feelings of contentment and well-being, and reduces stress.

19. Volunteer or Help Others:

Activity: Engage in acts of kindness by volunteering your time, helping a friend in need, or performing random acts of kindness for strangers.

Why It Works: Helping others promotes a sense of connection, purpose, and fulfillment, reducing stress and increasing feelings of well-being.

20. Practice Acceptance and Letting Go:

Activity: Practice acceptance of things you cannot change and let go of attachments to outcomes. Focus on what you can control and take proactive steps to address challenges.

Why It Works: Acceptance reduces resistance to reality, promotes inner peace, and reduces stress associated with trying to control or change things beyond your control.

Incorporate these additional tips into your daily routine to enhance relaxation, reduce stress, and promote overall well-being. Experiment with different strategies and find what works best for you. Remember that consistency is key, so make relaxation and stress reduction a regular part of your lifestyle.

Conclusion:

Incorporating these relaxation and stress reduction tips into your daily routine can help you manage stress more effectively, promote relaxation, and improve overall quality of life. Experiment with different techniques to find what works best for you, and remember to prioritize self-care regularly.

CHAPTER THREE

Nourishing Your Body and Mind

Fueling Your Body with Nutritious Foods

Fueling your body with nutritious foods is essential for overall health, energy levels, and well-being. Here are some tips for incorporating nutritious foods into your diet:

1. Prioritize Whole Foods:

Focus: Base your meals and snacks around whole, minimally processed foods such as fruits, vegetables, whole grains, lean proteins, and healthy fats.

Why It's Important: Whole foods are rich in essential nutrients, vitamins, minerals, and antioxidants, providing the body with the fuel it needs to function optimally.

2. Eat a Variety of Colorful Fruits and Vegetables:

Selection: Aim to include a diverse range of fruits and vegetables in your diet, focusing on different colors and types.

Why It's Important: Different-colored fruits and vegetables contain unique phytonutrients and antioxidants that offer various health benefits, such as reducing inflammation and supporting immune function.

3. Include Lean Proteins:

Sources: Incorporate lean protein sources into your meals, such as poultry, fish, tofu, beans, lentils, and Greek yogurt.

Why It's Important: Protein is essential for building and repairing tissues, supporting muscle growth, and maintaining a healthy metabolism.

4. Choose Whole Grains:

Selection: Opt for whole grains such as brown rice, quinoa, oats, barley, and whole wheat bread and pasta instead of refined grains.

Why It's Important: Whole grains are rich in fiber, vitamins, and minerals, providing sustained energy and promoting digestive health.

5. Incorporate Healthy Fats:

Sources: Include sources of healthy fats in your diet, such as avocados, nuts, seeds, olive oil, and fatty fish like salmon and mackerel.

Why It's Important: Healthy fats are essential for brain health, hormone production, and the absorption of fat-soluble vitamins.

6. Stay Hydrated:

Hydration: Drink plenty of water throughout the day and limit sugary drinks, sodas, and excessive caffeine intake.

Why It's Important: Proper hydration is essential for maintaining bodily functions, regulating body temperature, and supporting overall health and well-being.

7. Practice Portion Control:

Serving Sizes: Be mindful of portion sizes and avoid oversized servings, especially of high-calorie or high-fat foods.

Why It's Important: Practicing portion control helps prevent overeating, promotes weight management, and ensures a balanced intake of nutrients.

8. Limit Added Sugars and Processed Foods:

Reading Labels: Check food labels for added sugars and ingredients you can't pronounce. Limit consumption of processed foods, sugary snacks, and desserts.

Why It's Important: Excessive consumption of added sugars and processed foods is linked to various health issues, including obesity, diabetes, and heart disease.

9. Plan and Prepare Meals:

Meal Planning: Take time to plan and prepare meals ahead of time, focusing on nutritious, balanced options.

Why It's Important: Meal planning helps you make healthier choices, saves time and money, and reduces the likelihood of relying on unhealthy convenience foods.

10. Listen to Your Body:

Intuitive Eating: Pay attention to hunger and fullness cues, and eat mindfully without distractions.

Why It's Important: Listening to your body's signals helps prevent overeating, promotes a healthy relationship with food, and allows you to honor your body's needs.

By incorporating these tips into your dietary habits, you can fuel your body with the nutrients it needs to thrive, maintain energy levels, and support overall health and well-being. Remember that small, sustainable changes over time can lead to significant improvements in your diet and overall health.

Here's a breakdown of some nutritious foods you can incorporate into your diet across different food groups:

Fruits:

Berries: Blueberries, strawberries, raspberries, and blackberries are packed with antioxidants and vitamins.

Citrus Fruits: Oranges, lemons, grapefruits, and limes are rich in vitamin C and other nutrients.

Bananas: A great source of potassium and fiber, bananas are convenient and versatile.

Apples: High in fiber and antioxidants, apples make for a crunchy and satisfying snack.

Vegetables:

Leafy Greens: Spinach, kale, Swiss chard, and collard greens are nutrient powerhouses rich in vitamins, minerals, and antioxidants.

Cruciferous Vegetables: Broccoli, cauliflower, Brussels sprouts, and cabbage are high in fiber and cancer-fighting compounds.

Root Vegetables: Sweet potatoes, carrots, beets, and parsnips are rich in vitamins, minerals, and fiber.

Bell Peppers: Red, yellow, and green bell peppers are excellent sources of vitamin C and antioxidants.

Protein Sources:

Lean Poultry: Skinless chicken breast and turkey are low in fat and high in protein.

Fish: Salmon, tuna, mackerel, and sardines are rich in omega-3 fatty acids and protein.

Legumes: Beans, lentils, chickpeas, and peas are plant-based sources of protein, fiber, and essential nutrients.

Tofu and Tempeh: Soy-based products like tofu and tempeh are complete sources of protein and versatile in cooking.

Whole Grains:

Quinoa: A complete protein, quinoa is also high in fiber and various vitamins and minerals.

Brown Rice: High in fiber and rich in nutrients, brown rice is a healthy alternative to refined grains.

Oats: Oats are packed with fiber, particularly beta-glucan, which supports heart health.

Whole Wheat: Choose whole wheat bread, pasta, and crackers for added fiber and nutrients compared to refined grains.

Healthy Fats:

Avocado: Rich in monounsaturated fats, avocados are also a good source of fiber and potassium.

Nuts and Seeds: Almonds, walnuts, chia seeds, flaxseeds, and hemp seeds are nutritious sources of healthy fats, protein, and fiber.

Olive Oil: Extra virgin olive oil is rich in monounsaturated fats and antioxidants, making it a heart-healthy choice for cooking and dressing salads.

Fatty Fish: Salmon, trout, and mackerel are high in omega-3 fatty acids, which support brain health and reduce inflammation.

Dairy and Alternatives:

Greek Yogurt: High in protein and probiotics, Greek yogurt is a nutritious option for breakfast or snacks.

Almond Milk: A dairy-free alternative rich in vitamin E and calcium, almond milk is low in calories and suitable for those with lactose intolerance.

Cottage Cheese: Low in fat and high in protein, cottage cheese is a versatile ingredient for savory and sweet dishes.

Kefir: A fermented dairy product, kefir is rich in probiotics that support gut health and immune function.

Incorporating a variety of these nutritious foods into your diet can help provide essential nutrients, support overall health, and contribute to a balanced and satisfying eating pattern. Remember to prioritize whole, minimally processed foods and listen to your body's hunger and fullness cues.

The Role of Exercise in Energy Restoration

Exercise plays a crucial role in energy restoration by promoting physical and mental well-being through various mechanisms:

1. Increased Energy Levels:

Improved Circulation: Exercise enhances blood flow, delivering oxygen and nutrients to cells throughout the body, which boosts energy levels.

Release of Endorphins: Physical activity triggers the release of endorphins, neurotransmitters that reduce pain perception and promote feelings of euphoria and energy.

2. Stress Reduction:

Release of Tension: Exercise helps relieve physical tension in muscles, releasing pent-up stress and promoting relaxation.

Reduction of Cortisol: Regular exercise decreases levels of the stress hormone cortisol, which can otherwise contribute to fatigue and burnout.

3. Enhanced Mood and Mental Clarity:

Brain Function: Exercise stimulates the release of neurotransmitters like dopamine and serotonin, which improve mood, focus, and cognitive function.

Mind-Body Connection: Physical activity fosters a stronger mind-body connection, helping individuals feel more grounded, centered, and mentally clear.

4. Improved Sleep Quality:

Regulation of Sleep Patterns: Regular exercise helps regulate circadian rhythms and promote deeper, more restorative sleep, which contributes to overall energy restoration.

Reduction of Insomnia: Exercise can alleviate symptoms of insomnia and sleep disturbances, leading to better sleep quality and increased daytime energy.

5. Stress Resilience:

Building Resilience: Regular physical activity strengthens the body's ability to cope with stress, increasing resilience and reducing the impact of stress-related fatigue.

Emotional Well-being: Exercise provides a healthy outlet for processing emotions, reducing anxiety, and promoting a sense of well-being, which supports energy restoration.

6. Enhanced Physical Fitness:

Improved Endurance: Regular exercise improves cardiovascular health, endurance, and stamina, allowing individuals to perform daily activities with less fatigue.

Increased Strength and Flexibility: Strength training and flexibility exercises enhance muscular strength and joint mobility, reducing physical fatigue and promoting energy restoration.

7. Social Connection and Support:

Group Activities: Participating in exercise classes, team sports, or group fitness activities fosters social connection, camaraderie, and support, which can boost mood and energy levels.

Accountability: Exercising with a workout buddy or joining a community of like-minded individuals provides accountability and motivation to stay consistent with physical activity.

8. Overall Well-being:

Holistic Health: Regular exercise contributes to overall physical, mental, and emotional well-being, creating a foundation for sustained energy restoration and vitality.

Self-care: Prioritizing exercise as part of a self-care routine demonstrates a commitment to one's health and happiness, leading to greater energy and fulfillment in daily life.

By incorporating regular exercise into their routine, individuals can reap the numerous benefits that support energy restoration, resilience to stress, and overall well-being. Whether it's a brisk walk, a yoga session, or a gym workout, finding activities that they enjoy and that align with their preferences and abilities is key to maintaining a consistent exercise regimen.

Cultivating Mental Well-being through Mindfulness and Meditation

Cultivating mental well-being through mindfulness and meditation is a powerful practice that can have profound effects on overall health and happiness. Here's how mindfulness and meditation contribute to mental well-being:

1. Increased Awareness:

Mindfulness: Practicing mindfulness involves paying attention to the present moment without judgment. It helps individuals become more aware of their thoughts, emotions, and physical sensations, fostering a deeper understanding of themselves and their experiences.

2. Stress Reduction:

Stress Management: Mindfulness and meditation techniques help individuals develop skills to manage stress more effectively. By bringing attention to the present moment, individuals can cultivate a sense of calm and relaxation, reducing the impact of stress on mental and physical well-being.

3. Improved Emotional Regulation:

Emotional Resilience: Mindfulness and meditation practices strengthen the ability to regulate emotions and respond to challenges with greater equanimity. By cultivating a non-reactive stance towards difficult emotions, individuals can navigate life's ups and downs with more ease and grace.

4. Enhanced Focus and Concentration:

Attention Training: Meditation involves training the mind to focus and sustain attention on a chosen object, such as the breath or a mantra. This enhances concentration and cognitive function, leading to improved productivity and performance in various areas of life.

5. Greater Self-Compassion:

Kindness and Compassion: Mindfulness practices encourage self-compassion and self-acceptance. By cultivating a gentle and compassionate attitude towards oneself, individuals can reduce self-criticism and enhance feelings of worthiness and well-being.

6. Improved Sleep Quality:

Sleep Hygiene: Mindfulness techniques promote relaxation and stress reduction, which can improve sleep quality. By practicing mindfulness before bedtime, individuals can calm the mind and body, facilitating a more restful night's sleep.

7. Enhanced Resilience:

Adaptability: Mindfulness and meditation help individuals develop resilience to life's challenges. By cultivating a mindset of acceptance and non-judgment, individuals can bounce back more quickly from setbacks and setbacks, fostering greater emotional strength and flexibility.

8. Better Relationships:

Interpersonal Connection: Mindfulness practices enhance interpersonal relationships by promoting empathy, compassion, and active listening. By being fully present with others, individuals can strengthen connections and deepen understanding in their relationships.

9. Reduced Symptoms of Anxiety and Depression:

Mental Health: Mindfulness-based interventions have been shown to reduce symptoms of anxiety and depression. By cultivating present-moment awareness and acceptance, individuals can alleviate psychological distress and promote mental well-being.

10. Greater Overall Well-being:

Holistic Health: Mindfulness and meditation contribute to holistic well-being by nurturing the mind, body, and spirit. By integrating these practices into daily life, individuals can experience greater balance, harmony, and fulfillment.

By incorporating mindfulness and meditation into their daily routine, individuals can cultivate mental well-being and resilience, leading to greater happiness, peace, and fulfillment in life. Whether it's a formal meditation practice or informal mindfulness exercises, finding what resonates and committing to consistent practice is key to reaping the benefits of these transformative practices.

Mental well-being encompasses a state of overall psychological health and resilience, characterized by a sense of contentment, fulfillment, and emotional stability. Here are some key aspects and indicators of mental well-being:

1. Emotional Resilience:

Adaptability: The ability to cope with life's challenges and setbacks in a healthy and constructive manner.

Optimism: Maintaining a positive outlook on life, even in the face of adversity, and believing in one's ability to overcome obstacles.

2. Self-Awareness:

Mindfulness: Being aware of one's thoughts, feelings, and bodily sensations in the present moment without judgment.

Self-Reflection: Taking time for introspection and self-exploration to gain insight into one's values, beliefs, and behaviors.

3. Healthy Relationships:

Social Connection: Cultivating supportive relationships with friends, family, and community members that provide emotional support and companionship.

Boundaries: Setting and maintaining healthy boundaries in relationships to protect one's well-being and foster mutual respect.

4. Coping Strategies:

Effective Coping: Utilizing adaptive coping mechanisms to manage stress, regulate emotions, and problem-solve effectively.

Seeking Support: Knowing when to reach out for help from trusted individuals, such as friends, family, or mental health professionals, when needed.

5. Purpose and Meaning:

Sense of Purpose: Feeling a sense of direction and meaning in life, often derived from pursuing meaningful goals, passions, or values.

Personal Growth: Engaging in activities that promote personal development, learning, and self-improvement.

6. Psychological Well-being:

Positive Emotions: Experiencing a range of positive emotions such as joy, gratitude, and contentment, which contribute to overall well-being.

Resilience to Stress: Being able to effectively manage stressors and bounce back from adversity without significant long-term negative effects on mental health.

7. Self-Care:

Prioritizing Wellness: Engaging in activities that nurture physical, emotional, and spiritual well-being, such as exercise, relaxation, hobbies, and adequate sleep.

Setting Boundaries: Establishing limits on work, social commitments, and other responsibilities to prevent burnout and prioritize self-care.

8. Emotional Regulation:

Emotional Balance: Developing skills to regulate emotions and manage both positive and negative feelings in a healthy and adaptive way.

Mindfulness Practices: Incorporating mindfulness meditation, deep breathing exercises, and other relaxation techniques to promote emotional regulation and reduce stress.

9. Acceptance and Self-Compassion:

Self-Acceptance: Embracing oneself with kindness and compassion, including acceptance of strengths, weaknesses, and imperfections.

Non-Judgment: Cultivating a non-judgmental attitude towards oneself and others, allowing for greater self-compassion and empathy.

10. Fulfillment and Satisfaction:

Life Satisfaction: Feeling satisfied with one's life as a whole, including aspects such as work, relationships, health, and personal growth.

Gratitude: Cultivating a sense of gratitude for the present moment and appreciating the blessings and opportunities in one's life.

Conclusion:

Mental well-being is a multifaceted concept that encompasses various dimensions of psychological health, resilience, and fulfillment. By nurturing these aspects and adopting healthy habits and coping strategies, individuals can enhance their mental well-being and experience greater happiness, meaning, and overall quality of life.

CHAPTER FOUR

Unplugging and Reconnecting

Detoxifying from Digital Overload

Detoxifying from digital overload is crucial for maintaining mental well-being and finding balance in today's digital age. Here are some strategies to help you disconnect and reclaim control over your digital habits:

1. Set Clear Boundaries:

Designate Tech-Free Times: Establish specific times during the day when you will disconnect from digital devices, such as during meals, before bedtime, or during designated "unplugged" hours.

Create No-Tech Zones: Designate certain areas in your home, such as the bedroom or dining area, as tech-free zones to promote relaxation and connection with others.

2. Limit Screen Time:

Use Screen Time Tracking: Monitor and limit your daily screen time using built-in features on your devices or third-party apps. Set goals for reducing screen time gradually to avoid overwhelm.

Schedule Breaks: Incorporate regular breaks from screens throughout the day, such as every hour, to rest your eyes and recharge your mind.

3. Practice Digital Detox Activities:

Engage in Offline Hobbies: Rediscover offline activities that bring you joy and fulfillment, such as reading books, gardening, cooking, or playing musical instruments.

Spend Time in Nature: Disconnect from digital devices and spend time outdoors, enjoying activities like hiking, walking, or simply sitting in a park.

4. Establish Tech-Free Rituals:

Morning Routine: Start your day without immediately checking your phone or emails. Begin with a mindful activity such as meditation, stretching, or journaling to set a positive tone for the day.

Evening Wind-Down: Create a calming bedtime routine that doesn't involve screens, such as reading a book, taking a bath, or practicing relaxation techniques.

5. Prioritize Real-Life Connections:

Face-to-Face Interaction: Make time for in-person connections with friends, family, and loved ones. Schedule social activities or outings where digital devices are minimized or set aside.

Quality Time: Spend quality time with loved ones without distractions from digital devices. Engage in meaningful conversations, games, or activities that foster connection and intimacy.

6. Practice Mindfulness:

Mindful Technology Use: Cultivate awareness of your digital habits and their impact on your well-being. Practice mindful use of technology by checking in with yourself before reaching for your devices.

Mindfulness Meditation: Incorporate mindfulness meditation into your routine to develop greater awareness, focus, and emotional regulation, helping you navigate digital overload more effectively.

7. Set Digital Boundaries:

Manage Notifications: Disable non-essential notifications on your devices to minimize distractions and interruptions throughout the day.

Establish Communication Boundaries: Set boundaries around your availability for emails, messages, and calls to prevent constant connectivity and create space for offline activities.

8. Practice Self-Care:

Physical Activity: Engage in regular physical exercise to reduce stress, boost mood, and counteract the sedentary nature of prolonged screen time.

Healthy Habits: Prioritize self-care activities such as adequate sleep, healthy eating, and stress management techniques to support overall well-being and resilience.

9. Seek Support:

Accountability Partner: Partner with a friend or family member to support each other in reducing screen time and practicing digital detox together.

Professional Help: If digital overload significantly impacts your mental health and well-being, consider seeking support from a mental health professional who can provide guidance and strategies for managing digital habits.

10. Reflect and Adjust:

Regular Evaluation: Reflect on your digital habits regularly and assess their impact on your mental and emotional well-being. Adjust your strategies and boundaries as needed to find a balance that works for you.

Celebrate Progress: Acknowledge and celebrate small victories in reducing screen time and practicing digital detox, recognizing the positive impact on your overall well-being.

By implementing these strategies and prioritizing intentional digital use, you can detoxify from digital overload and create space for greater presence, connection, and well-being in your life. Remember that finding balance is a continual process, so be patient and compassionate with yourself as you navigate your digital detox journey.

Unplugging and reconnecting with yourself, others, and the world around you is essential for maintaining balance and well-being in today's hyper-connected world. Here are some tips to help you unplug and foster meaningful connections:

1. Set Clear Boundaries:

Define Tech-Free Times: Establish specific times during the day or week when you will disconnect from digital devices. This could include evenings, weekends, or certain hours during the day.

Create Tech-Free Zones: Designate areas in your home, such as the dining room or bedroom, where digital devices are not allowed to promote relaxation and interpersonal connection.

2. Engage in Offline Activities:

Rediscover Hobbies: Spend time engaging in activities that you enjoy and that don't involve screens, such as reading, cooking, painting, or gardening.

Outdoor Adventures: Spend time outdoors exploring nature, going for walks or hikes, or simply enjoying the beauty of the natural world.

3. Prioritize Face-to-Face Interaction:

Quality Time with Loved Ones: Make an effort to spend uninterrupted quality time with family and friends. Plan activities or outings where you can connect and bond without digital distractions.

Social Gatherings: Host or attend social gatherings where digital devices are minimized, allowing for more meaningful conversations and connections.

4. Practice Mindfulness and Presence:

Mindful Awareness: Cultivate mindfulness by paying attention to the present moment without judgment. Practice mindfulness meditation or simply engage fully in whatever you are doing, whether it's eating, walking, or talking to someone.

Digital Mindfulness: When you do use digital devices, practice mindfulness by being intentional and present. Limit multitasking and distractions, and focus on one task at a time.

5. Nurture Self-Care:

Unwind and Relax: Take time for self-care activities that promote relaxation and well-being, such as taking a bath, practicing yoga or meditation, or listening to music.

Disconnect Before Bed: Create a bedtime routine that doesn't involve screens to promote better sleep quality and relaxation. Engage in calming activities such as reading or journaling before bedtime.

6. Foster Meaningful Connections:

Deep Conversations: Engage in meaningful conversations with friends and loved ones, sharing thoughts, feelings, and experiences openly and authentically.

Express Gratitude: Take time to express gratitude for the people in your life and the experiences you have shared together. Cultivate an attitude of appreciation and connection.

7. Reconnect with Nature:

Nature Walks: Spend time in nature connecting with the environment around you. Go for walks in the park, hike in the mountains, or visit the beach to recharge and rejuvenate.

Outdoor Activities: Engage in outdoor activities such as gardening, birdwatching, or stargazing to connect with the natural world and experience its beauty.

8. Practice Active Listening:

Be Present: Practice active listening when interacting with others, giving them your full attention and showing genuine interest in what they have to say.

Validate Emotions: Validate the emotions of others and offer support and empathy when needed. Create a safe space for open and honest communication.

9. Embrace Solitude:

Me Time: Spend time alone engaging in activities that nourish your soul and recharge your energy. Enjoy moments of solitude for reflection, creativity, and self-discovery.

Disconnect to Reconnect: Disconnect from digital devices periodically to create space for introspection and self-awareness. Use this time to reconnect with yourself and your inner wisdom.

10. Reflect and Appreciate:

Reflect on Your Values: Take time to reflect on your values, priorities, and what matters most to you in life. Align your actions with your values to live a more purposeful and fulfilling life.

Appreciate the Moment: Practice gratitude for the simple joys and pleasures of everyday life. Cultivate an attitude of appreciation and presence, savoring each moment fully.

By unplugging from digital distractions and reconnecting with yourself, others, and the world around you, you can cultivate deeper connections, enhance well-being, and experience greater fulfillment and meaning in life. Remember that finding balance is a continual process, so be gentle with yourself as you navigate your journey of unplugging and reconnecting.

Finding Balance in a Hyperconnected World

Finding balance in a hyperconnected world is essential for maintaining mental well-being, productivity, and overall quality of life. Here are some strategies to help you achieve balance:

1. Set Boundaries:

Establish Tech-Free Times: Designate specific times during the day when you disconnect from digital devices, such as during meals, before bedtime, or during leisure activities.

Create No-Tech Zones: Designate certain areas in your home, such as the bedroom or dining area, as tech-free zones to promote relaxation and interpersonal connection.

2. Prioritize Tasks:

Practice Time Management: Prioritize tasks and allocate specific time slots for work, leisure, and self-care activities. Use time-blocking techniques to schedule focused work periods and breaks throughout the day.

Set Realistic Goals: Set realistic and achievable goals for yourself, both personally and professionally. Break larger tasks into smaller, manageable steps to avoid feeling overwhelmed.

3. Practice Mindfulness:

Be Present: Cultivate mindfulness by bringing your attention to the present moment without judgment. Practice mindfulness meditation or engage fully in whatever activity you are doing, whether it's work, exercise, or spending time with loved ones.

Digital Mindfulness: Practice mindfulness when using digital devices by being intentional and present. Limit multitasking and distractions, and focus on one task at a time to improve focus and productivity.

4. Nurture Relationships:

Quality Time: Make time for meaningful connections with family and friends. Prioritize face-to-face interactions and engage in activities that foster connection and intimacy.

Communication: Communicate openly and honestly with loved ones about your need for balance and boundaries. Set aside dedicated time for quality conversations and shared experiences.

5. Manage Digital Consumption:

Limit Screen Time: Set limits on your daily screen time and prioritize offline activities that promote well-being and connection.

Curate Your Digital Environment: Regularly review and declutter your digital devices, including emails, apps, and social media accounts. Unsubscribe from unnecessary notifications and unsubscribe from apps or services that no longer serve your needs.

6. Practice Self-Care:

Prioritize Well-Being: Take care of your physical, mental, and emotional well-being by engaging in self-care activities that nourish your body and soul.

Set Aside Me Time: Schedule regular downtime for relaxation and rejuvenation. Engage in activities that bring you joy and replenish your energy, such as reading, practicing hobbies, or taking a bath.

7. Embrace Flexibility:

Be Adaptive: Be open to adjusting your routines and schedules as needed to accommodate unexpected changes or priorities.

Learn to Say No: Set boundaries and learn to say no to commitments or requests that don't align with your priorities or values. Focus on what truly matters to you and let go of unnecessary obligations.

8. Seek Support:

Reach Out: Don't hesitate to seek support from friends, family, or professionals if you're feeling overwhelmed or struggling to find balance.

Join Communities: Connect with like-minded individuals who share your values and goals for finding balance in a hyperconnected world. Join online or offline communities for support, encouragement, and accountability.

9. Reflect and Adjust:

Regular Evaluation: Take time to reflect on your current lifestyle and assess whether it aligns with your goals and values. Make adjustments as needed to prioritize balance and well-being.

Celebrate Progress: Acknowledge and celebrate your successes and achievements along the way. Recognize the steps you've taken towards finding balance and continue to strive for growth and improvement.

10. Cultivate Gratitude:

Practice Gratitude: Cultivate an attitude of gratitude for the blessings and opportunities in your life, both big and small. Take time each day to reflect on what you're grateful for and express appreciation to others.

Focus on What Matters: Keep perspective on what truly matters to you and prioritize your time and energy accordingly. Let go of comparison and embrace the uniqueness of your journey towards balance and fulfillment.

By implementing these strategies and prioritizing balance in your life, you can navigate the challenges of living in a hyperconnected world while nurturing your well-being and cultivating a sense of fulfillment and purpose. Remember that finding balance is an ongoing process, and it's okay to adjust and refine your approach as needed to better align with your values and goals.

Living in a hyperconnected world means being constantly surrounded by technology and interconnected systems that shape various aspects of our lives. Here are some examples of how this hyperconnectivity manifests in different domains:

1. Communication:

Social Media Platforms: Platforms like Facebook, Instagram, Twitter, and LinkedIn enable instant communication and connection with friends, family, colleagues, and acquaintances around the world.

Messaging Apps: Apps such as WhatsApp, Messenger, and WeChat facilitate real-time messaging, voice calls, and video chats, allowing people to stay in touch regardless of geographical distance.

2. Information Access:

Search Engines: Platforms like Google, Bing, and Yahoo provide access to vast amounts of information on virtually any topic, empowering individuals to find answers to their questions and solve problems quickly.

Online Encyclopedias: Websites like Wikipedia offer a wealth of knowledge contributed by users worldwide, serving as a go-to resource for academic research, general inquiries, and learning.

3. Entertainment:

Streaming Services: Platforms such as Netflix, Amazon Prime Video, Hulu, and Disney+ allow users to stream movies, TV shows, documentaries, and other content on-demand, anytime and anywhere.

Gaming Communities: Online gaming platforms like Xbox Live, PlayStation Network, and Steam connect gamers worldwide, enabling multiplayer gaming experiences and social interaction.

4. Work and Productivity:

Remote Work Tools: Platforms like Zoom, Microsoft Teams, and Slack facilitate remote collaboration, video conferencing, file sharing, and project management, enabling flexible work arrangements and global teamwork.

Cloud Computing: Services such as Google Workspace, Microsoft 365, and Dropbox provide cloud-based storage, document collaboration, and productivity tools, allowing users to access and work on files from any device with an internet connection.

5. E-Commerce:

Online Marketplaces: Websites and apps like Amazon, eBay, and Alibaba offer a vast array of products and services for purchase, with features such as one-click ordering, personalized recommendations, and fast shipping.

Digital Payments: Platforms such as PayPal, Venmo, Apple Pay, and Google Pay enable secure and convenient digital transactions, making it easy to send and receive money online.

6. Transportation and Navigation:

Ride-Hailing Apps: Services like Uber, Lyft, and Grab provide on-demand transportation options, allowing users to book rides, track drivers, and pay fares seamlessly through mobile apps.

GPS Navigation: Apps like Google Maps, Waze, and Apple Maps offer real-time navigation and traffic information, helping users navigate unfamiliar routes and optimize travel times.

7. Health and Fitness:

Wearable Devices: Smartwatches, fitness trackers, and health monitors like Fitbit, Apple Watch, and Garmin track physical activity, monitor vital signs, and provide insights into health and fitness goals.

Telehealth Services: Platforms such as Doctor On Demand, Teladoc, and Amwell offer remote healthcare consultations, diagnoses, and prescriptions, expanding access to medical care and support.

8. Smart Home Technology:

Voice Assistants: Devices like Amazon Echo (Alexa), Google Home, and Apple HomePod enable voice-controlled operation of smart home devices, entertainment systems, and virtual assistants.

Smart Appliances: IoT-enabled appliances such as smart thermostats, lighting systems, security cameras, and kitchen gadgets allow remote monitoring and control via smartphone apps or voice commands.

9. Social Movements and Activism:

Online Advocacy: Social media platforms and digital campaigns amplify voices, raise awareness, and mobilize support for social justice causes, environmental activism, and political movements.

Crowdfunding Platforms: Websites like GoFundMe, Kickstarter, and Indiegogo enable individuals and organizations to raise funds for charitable causes, creative projects, and entrepreneurial ventures.

10. Education and Learning:

Online Learning Platforms: Websites and apps like Coursera, Udemy, Khan Academy, and Duolingo offer a wide range of courses, tutorials, and resources for lifelong learning and skill development.

Virtual Classrooms: Remote learning platforms and video conferencing tools facilitate online education, virtual classrooms, and distance learning programs for students of all ages.

These examples illustrate the pervasive influence of technology and interconnected systems in our daily lives, shaping how we communicate, work, socialize, learn, and engage with the world around us in a hyperconnected society.

Reconnecting with Nature and the Present Moment

Reconnecting with nature and the present moment is essential for promoting mental well-being, reducing stress, and fostering a sense of peace and connection with the world around us. Here are some strategies to help you cultivate this reconnection:

1. Spend Time Outdoors:

Nature Walks: Take leisurely walks in natural settings such as parks, forests, or beaches. Pay attention to the sights, sounds, and sensations of the natural environment around you.

Hiking: Explore hiking trails or nature reserves to immerse yourself in the beauty of nature and experience the serenity of remote landscapes.

2. Practice Mindful Awareness:

Mindful Walking: Practice mindful walking by focusing on each step and sensation as you move. Notice the feeling of your feet touching the ground and the rhythm of your breath.

Nature Meditation: Find a quiet spot outdoors to sit or lie down comfortably. Close your eyes and tune into the sounds, smells, and sensations of nature around you, allowing yourself to be fully present in the moment.

3. Engage Your Senses:

Nature Observation: Take time to observe and appreciate the details of the natural world, such as the colors of flowers, the textures of tree bark, or the patterns of clouds in the sky.

Listen to Nature: Tune into the sounds of birds singing, leaves rustling in the wind, or water flowing in a stream. Allow these natural sounds to calm your mind and ground you in the present moment.

4. Disconnect from Digital Distractions:

Tech-Free Time: Set aside dedicated time each day to disconnect from digital devices and immerse yourself in nature. Turn off your phone or put it on airplane mode to minimize distractions.

Digital Detox: Take occasional breaks from technology by unplugging from screens and spending time outdoors without any electronic devices.

5. Practice Gratitude:

Nature Appreciation: Cultivate gratitude for the beauty and abundance of nature by acknowledging the gifts it provides, such as clean air, fresh water, and stunning landscapes.

Gratitude Journaling: Keep a journal where you write down things you are grateful for in nature, such as a colorful sunset, a fragrant flower, or a peaceful moment by the water.

6. Engage in Nature-Based Activities:

Gardening: Planting, tending to, and harvesting plants in a garden can be a meditative and rewarding way to connect with nature and experience the cycle of growth and renewal.

Outdoor Yoga or Tai Chi: Practice yoga or tai chi outdoors to connect mind, body, and spirit with the natural elements and energy of the environment.

7. Foster Connection with Wildlife:

Birdwatching: Set up a bird feeder in your yard or visit local parks and nature reserves to observe and identify different bird species. Binoculars and a field guide can enhance your birdwatching experience.

Animal Encounters: Spend time observing animals in their natural habitats, such as squirrels, rabbits, or deer. Respect their space and observe from a distance to avoid disturbing them.

8. Cultivate a Nature-Inspired Mindset:

Nature Metaphors: Reflect on the lessons and wisdom that nature can offer, such as resilience in the face of adversity, adaptability to change, and the interconnectedness of all living things.

Nature-Inspired Creativity: Use nature as a source of inspiration for creative activities such as drawing, painting, photography, or writing poetry.

9. Practice Environmental Stewardship:

Leave No Trace: Practice responsible outdoor ethics by minimizing your impact on natural environments. Leave natural areas cleaner than you found them and follow Leave No Trace principles.

Sustainable Living: Adopt eco-friendly habits and lifestyle choices that reduce your carbon footprint and support environmental conservation efforts.

10. Share Nature Experiences with Others:

Outdoor Activities with Loved Ones: Invite friends, family members, or colleagues to join you for outdoor activities such as picnics, nature walks, or camping trips.

Nature-Based Education: Teach children and young people about the importance of nature and the benefits of spending time outdoors. Encourage them to explore and appreciate the natural world around them.

Reconnecting with nature and the present moment can bring a sense of calm, joy, and rejuvenation to your life. By incorporating these practices into your routine, you can cultivate a deeper connection with nature and experience the myriad benefits it offers for your physical, mental, and emotional well-being.

CHAPTER FIVE

Setting Boundaries and Prioritizing Self-Care

Establishing Healthy Boundaries in Relationships and Work

Establishing healthy boundaries is essential for maintaining balance, respect, and well-being in relationships and work settings. Here's how you can establish and maintain healthy boundaries in both areas:

1. Understand Your Needs and Limits:

Self-Awareness: Take time to reflect on your values, priorities, and personal limits. Identify what is important to you and what you need to feel comfortable and respected in relationships and work.

2. Communicate Clearly:

Express Your Needs: Clearly communicate your boundaries, expectations, and limitations to others in a calm and assertive manner. Use "I" statements to express your feelings and needs without blaming or criticizing.

Be Direct: Avoid assuming that others will automatically know your boundaries. Be direct and upfront about your boundaries to ensure mutual understanding and respect.

3. Learn to Say No:

Set Limits: Practice saying no to requests, obligations, or situations that do not align with your values, priorities, or well-being. It's okay to decline invitations or opportunities that feel overwhelming or draining.

Prioritize Yourself: Remember that setting boundaries and saying no is not selfish—it's an act of self-care and self-preservation.

4. Identify Red Flags:

Recognize Violations: Pay attention to situations or behaviors that violate your boundaries or make you feel uncomfortable, disrespected, or unsafe.

Trust Your Instincts: Trust your instincts and feelings. If something doesn't feel right, it's important to honor your intuition and take steps to protect yourself.

5. Establish Boundaries in Relationships:

Define Relationship Dynamics: Clarify expectations and boundaries within your relationships, whether they are with friends, family members, romantic partners, or colleagues.

Respect Each Other's Boundaries: Respect the boundaries of others and communicate openly about your own boundaries. Mutual respect and understanding are key to healthy relationships.

6. Set Boundaries at Work:

Clarify Expectations: Communicate with your supervisor, colleagues, and clients about your role, responsibilities, and availability. Establish clear boundaries around work hours, workload, and communication outside of work.

Protect Personal Time: Set boundaries to protect your personal time and prevent work from encroaching on your personal life. Establish limits on after-hours work emails, calls, and meetings.

7. Practice Self-Care:

Prioritize Well-Being: Make self-care a priority by engaging in activities that nourish your body, mind, and spirit. Set aside time for relaxation, hobbies, exercise, and socializing.

Recognize Burnout: Be vigilant for signs of burnout, such as exhaustion, irritability, and decreased productivity. Take proactive steps to prevent burnout by setting boundaries and practicing self-care.

8. Seek Support:

Talk to Others: Reach out to trusted friends, family members, or colleagues for support and guidance in establishing and maintaining healthy boundaries.

Therapy or Counseling: Consider seeking professional help from a therapist or counselor if you're struggling to set boundaries or assert yourself in relationships or work situations.

9. Be Consistent:

Follow Through: Once you've established boundaries, be consistent in enforcing them. Hold yourself and others accountable for respecting boundaries and maintaining healthy relationships and work dynamics.

Adjust as Needed: Be open to adjusting your boundaries as circumstances change or as you gain more clarity about your needs and limits.

10. Practice Empathy and Understanding:

Empathize with Others: Recognize that everyone has their own boundaries, needs, and challenges. Practice empathy and understanding when navigating relationships and work dynamics.

Communicate Respectfully: Approach boundary-setting with empathy and compassion, taking into account the feelings and perspectives of others while advocating for your own well-being.

By establishing healthy boundaries in relationships and work, you can cultivate more fulfilling connections, reduce stress, and create a greater sense of balance and well-being in your life. Remember that setting boundaries is a skill that takes practice and may require ongoing adjustments, but it's an essential aspect of self-care and personal growth.

Saying No with Confidence and Grace

Saying no with confidence and grace is an important skill that allows you to set boundaries, prioritize your needs, and maintain balance in your life. Here are some tips to help you say no assertively and respectfully:

1. Be Clear and Direct:

Use Clear Language: Say "no" directly and clearly without beating around the bush. Avoid using ambiguous or apologetic language that may leave room for misinterpretation.

State Your Reasons: Provide a brief explanation for why you are declining the request, if appropriate. You don't owe anyone a detailed explanation, but offering a brief reason can help clarify your decision.

2. Express Appreciation:

Acknowledge the Request: Express gratitude for the opportunity or invitation, even if you ultimately decide to decline it. Acknowledging the request shows that you value the relationship or opportunity.

Express Regret: Communicate your regret for not being able to accommodate the request at this time. Expressing regret acknowledges the other person's disappointment while affirming your decision.

3. Set Boundaries:

Know Your Limits: Be aware of your own limits, priorities, and commitments before agreeing to take on new tasks or obligations. Setting clear boundaries helps you avoid overcommitting yourself.

Be Firm: Stand firm in your decision to say no, even if the other person tries to persuade or guilt-trip you into changing your mind. Remember that it's okay to prioritize your own well-being and needs.

4. Offer Alternatives:

Provide Solutions: Offer alternative solutions or compromises, if possible, that may meet the other person's needs or address their concerns without compromising your own boundaries.

Refer to Someone Else: If you're unable to fulfill the request yourself, consider referring the person to someone else who may be better suited to help. This shows that you're still willing to assist in finding a solution.

5. Use Assertive Body Language:

Maintain Eye Contact: Make and maintain eye contact with the person you're speaking to. Eye contact conveys confidence and sincerity in your response.

Stand Tall: Stand or sit up straight with your shoulders back to convey confidence and assertiveness. Avoid crossing your arms, which can come across as defensive.

6. Practice Self-Care:

Prioritize Your Well-Being: Remember that it's important to prioritize your own well-being and needs. Saying no allows you to protect your time, energy, and resources for activities that are truly meaningful to you.

Practice Self-Compassion: Be kind to yourself and recognize that it's okay to say no. Practice self-compassion and remind yourself that setting boundaries is a healthy and necessary aspect of self-care.

7. Be Consistent:

Stay True to Your Boundaries: Be consistent in enforcing your boundaries and saying no when necessary. Consistency reinforces your credibility and helps others understand and respect your limits.

Don't Feel Guilty: Let go of any feelings of guilt or obligation associated with saying no. Remember that you're not responsible for meeting everyone else's needs and that it's okay to prioritize yourself.

8. Practice Saying No:

Role-Play Scenarios: Practice saying no in different scenarios with a friend, family member, or trusted colleague. Role-playing can help you become more comfortable and confident in asserting yourself.

Start Small: Begin by saying no to minor requests or obligations before tackling more significant or challenging ones. Building confidence gradually can make it easier to assert yourself in more demanding situations.

9. Reflect on Past Experiences:

Learn from Past Experiences: Reflect on past instances where you said yes when you wanted to say no. Consider what you could have done differently and apply those lessons to future situations.

Celebrate Your Successes: Acknowledge and celebrate your successes in setting boundaries and saying no. Recognize the progress you've made and the positive impact it has had on your well-being.

10. Seek Support:

Lean on Your Support System: Reach out to friends, family members, or mentors for encouragement and support as you work on saying no with confidence and grace.

Consider Professional Help: If you struggle with asserting yourself or setting boundaries, consider seeking guidance from a therapist or counselor who can provide strategies and support.

Remember that saying no is not a rejection of the person making the request but rather a affirmation of your own needs and boundaries. By saying no with confidence and grace, you empower yourself to live authentically and prioritize what truly matters to you.

Making Self-Care a Non-Negotiable Priority

Making self-care a non-negotiable priority is essential for maintaining your physical, mental, and emotional well-being. Here's how you can prioritize self-care and ensure it remains a central focus in your life:

1. Recognize the Importance of Self-Care:

Understand the Benefits: Educate yourself about the importance of self-care and the positive impact it can have on your overall health and quality of life.

Acknowledge Your Worth: Recognize that you deserve to prioritize your well-being and make self-care a non-negotiable aspect of your daily routine.

2. Define What Self-Care Means to You:

Identify Your Needs: Reflect on the activities and practices that nourish your body, mind, and spirit. Determine what self-care looks like for you personally.

Customize Your Routine: Tailor your self-care routine to fit your individual preferences, interests, and lifestyle. Focus on activities that bring you joy, relaxation, and rejuvenation.

3. Schedule Dedicated Self-Care Time:

Block Out Time: Set aside dedicated time in your schedule for self-care activities. Treat this time as non-negotiable, just like any other important commitment or obligation.

Prioritize Yourself: Make yourself a priority by scheduling self-care activities at times when you're most likely to follow through and fully engage in them.

4. Set Boundaries:

Protect Your Time: Establish boundaries to protect your self-care time from being infringed upon by other commitments or obligations.

Learn to Say No: Practice saying no to requests, invitations, or activities that conflict with your self-care priorities. Prioritize your well-being over people-pleasing or overcommitting.

5. Practice Mindfulness:

Be Present: Cultivate mindfulness by being fully present in the moment during your self-care activities. Focus on the sensations, thoughts, and emotions that arise without judgment.

Savor the Experience: Take time to savor and appreciate the benefits of self-care, whether it's the feeling of relaxation during a bath or the sense of accomplishment after a workout.

6. Create a Self-Care Toolkit:

Identify Resources: Compile a list of self-care activities, resources, and tools that you can turn to when you need a boost or are feeling stressed.

Include Variety: Include a variety of activities in your toolkit, such as exercise, meditation, creative hobbies, or spending time in nature, to address different aspects of your well-being.

7. Practice Self-Compassion:

Be Kind to Yourself: Practice self-compassion by treating yourself with the same kindness and understanding that you would offer to a friend in need.

Let Go of Perfectionism: Release the need to be perfect in your self-care practice. Embrace imperfection and allow yourself to enjoy the process without judgment.

8. Make Self-Care Enjoyable:

Choose Activities You Love: Select self-care activities that you genuinely enjoy and look forward to doing. Find pleasure and fulfillment in the process.

Get Creative: Explore new self-care practices and experiment with different activities to keep your routine fresh and exciting.

9. Enlist Support:

Involve Others: Share your self-care goals and priorities with friends, family members, or partners who can offer support, encouragement, and accountability.

Seek Professional Help: If you're struggling to prioritize self-care or maintain a consistent routine, consider seeking guidance from a therapist or counselor who can provide personalized support.

10. Celebrate Your Progress:

Acknowledge Your Achievements: Celebrate your successes and milestones in prioritizing self-care. Recognize the positive changes and improvements in your well-being.

Practice Gratitude: Express gratitude for the opportunity to care for yourself and invest in your health and happiness. Cultivate an attitude of appreciation for the gift of self-care.

By making self-care a non-negotiable priority in your life, you can nurture your physical, mental, and emotional well-being, increase resilience to stress, and cultivate a greater sense of balance and fulfillment. Remember that self-care is not selfish—it's essential for your overall health and happiness.

CHAPTER SIX

Cultivating Sustainable Habits for Long-Term Energy

Building Resilience through Consistent Habits

Building resilience through consistent habits is a powerful way to strengthen your ability to adapt and thrive in the face of adversity. Here are some key habits that can help you develop resilience:

1. Cultivate Self-Awareness:

Reflection: Take time to reflect on your thoughts, feelings, and reactions to challenging situations. Develop a deeper understanding of your strengths, weaknesses, and coping mechanisms.

Mindfulness Practice: Engage in mindfulness meditation or other mindfulness exercises to increase self-awareness and cultivate a non-judgmental awareness of the present moment.

2. Develop Positive Thinking:

Optimism: Cultivate an optimistic outlook by focusing on opportunities for growth and learning in difficult situations. Challenge negative thought patterns and reframe setbacks as temporary and surmountable.

Gratitude Practice: Practice gratitude by regularly reflecting on the things you're thankful for in your life. Gratitude can shift your perspective and increase resilience in the face of adversity.

3. Maintain Healthy Habits:

Physical Health: Prioritize regular exercise, nutritious eating, and adequate sleep to support your physical and mental well-being. Physical health is closely linked to resilience and coping ability.

Sleep Hygiene: Establish a consistent sleep routine and create a sleep-friendly environment to ensure restorative sleep. Quality sleep is essential for cognitive function, mood regulation, and stress management.

4. Foster Supportive Relationships:

Connection: Build and nurture strong relationships with family, friends, and community members. Seek support from others during times of stress and offer support to those in need.

Communication: Practice open and honest communication in your relationships. Express your needs and emotions effectively and listen empathetically to others.

5. Develop Problem-Solving Skills:

Adaptability: Embrace change and uncertainty as opportunities for growth. Develop the flexibility to adjust your goals and plans in response to new information or challenges.

Resourcefulness: Develop problem-solving skills and seek creative solutions to overcome obstacles. Break challenges down into manageable steps and take proactive action.

6. Set Goals and Take Action:

Goal Setting: Set realistic and achievable goals for yourself, both short-term and long-term. Goals provide direction and motivation, helping you stay focused and resilient in pursuit of your objectives.

Action Planning: Break down your goals into actionable steps and create a plan for achieving them. Take consistent action towards your goals, even in the face of setbacks or obstacles.

7. Practice Stress Management:

Stress Reduction Techniques: Incorporate stress management techniques into your daily routine, such as deep breathing exercises, progressive muscle relaxation, or guided imagery.

Self-Care: Prioritize self-care activities that promote relaxation and well-being, such as spending time in nature, engaging in hobbies, or practicing mindfulness.

8. Foster a Growth Mindset:

Learning Orientation: Embrace challenges as opportunities for learning and growth. Adopt a growth mindset that views setbacks as temporary setbacks rather than permanent failures.

Resilience Narratives: Reflect on past experiences of resilience and draw inspiration from your ability to overcome adversity. Use these narratives to reinforce your belief in your capacity for resilience.

9. Seek Meaning and Purpose:

Values Clarification: Reflect on your core values and what gives your life meaning and purpose. Align your goals and actions with your values to create a sense of meaning and fulfillment.

Service and Contribution: Find ways to contribute to something greater than yourself, whether through volunteer work, advocacy, or acts of kindness. Connecting to a sense of purpose can enhance resilience.

10. Practice Self-Compassion:

Kindness Toward Yourself: Treat yourself with kindness, compassion, and understanding, especially during times of difficulty or failure. Practice self-compassion by offering yourself the same care and support you would offer to a friend.

Emotional Regulation: Develop healthy emotional regulation skills to manage difficult emotions effectively. Allow yourself to experience and express your feelings while maintaining perspective and self-control.

Consistency is key when it comes to building resilience through habits. By integrating these practices into your daily life and maintaining them over time, you can strengthen your resilience and increase your capacity to navigate life's challenges with courage, adaptability, and inner strength.

Creating a Supportive Environment for Energy Renewal

Creating a supportive environment for energy renewal is essential for maintaining vitality, productivity, and overall well-being. Here are some strategies to help you cultivate an environment that promotes energy renewal:

1. Designate Restful Spaces:

Create Relaxation Zones: Designate specific areas in your home or workplace for relaxation and rejuvenation. Choose quiet, comfortable spaces with minimal distractions where you can unwind and recharge.

Comfortable Seating: Invest in ergonomic furniture and cozy seating options, such as plush chairs or cushions, to enhance comfort and relaxation in your designated restful spaces.

2. Prioritize Natural Light and Fresh Air:

Maximize Natural Light: Position furniture and workspaces near windows to maximize exposure to natural light. Natural light can boost mood, energy levels, and overall well-being.

Ventilation: Ensure proper ventilation and airflow in indoor spaces by opening windows or using air purifiers. Fresh air can improve air quality and help reduce feelings of fatigue and sluggishness.

3. Incorporate Nature Elements:

Indoor Plants: Bring nature indoors by incorporating plants into your environment. Indoor plants not only add beauty and greenery but also help purify the air and create a calming atmosphere.

Natural Materials: Choose furnishings and decor made from natural materials such as wood, stone, or bamboo to create a sense of connection to the natural world.

4. Establish Healthy Work Practices:

Work-Life Balance: Set boundaries between work and personal life to avoid burnout and maintain energy levels. Establish specific work hours and designate time for rest, relaxation, and leisure activities.

Regular Breaks: Take regular breaks throughout the day to rest and recharge. Use breaks to engage in brief relaxation exercises, stretch, or step outside for fresh air and a change of scenery.

5. Foster Supportive Relationships:

Social Connection: Cultivate supportive relationships with family, friends, and colleagues who uplift and energize you. Prioritize quality time spent with loved ones and seek social support when needed.

Positive Communication: Foster open, honest, and supportive communication in your relationships. Surround yourself with people who encourage and validate your feelings and experiences.

6. Encourage Movement and Exercise:

Active Breaks: Incorporate movement into your daily routine by taking short walks, stretching, or practicing yoga during breaks. Physical activity boosts energy levels and promotes mental clarity.

Fitness Opportunities: Create opportunities for exercise and physical activity by joining a gym, taking fitness classes, or participating in outdoor recreational activities that you enjoy.

7. Practice Stress Reduction Techniques:

Stress Management: Develop stress reduction techniques such as deep breathing exercises, meditation, or mindfulness practices to promote relaxation and calmness.

Mindfulness Moments: Incorporate mindfulness into your daily life by pausing to focus on the present moment and engage your senses. Mindfulness can help reduce stress and increase energy levels.

8. Prioritize Sleep:

Sleep Environment: Create a conducive sleep environment that is dark, quiet, and comfortable. Invest in a supportive mattress and pillows to promote restful sleep and prevent discomfort.

Sleep Hygiene: Establish a consistent sleep routine and practice good sleep hygiene habits, such as avoiding screens before bedtime, limiting caffeine intake, and creating a relaxing bedtime ritual.

9. Nourish Your Body:

Healthy Nutrition: Prioritize nutritious foods that fuel your body and provide sustained energy throughout the day. Incorporate a balance of whole grains, fruits, vegetables, lean proteins, and healthy fats into your diet.

Hydration: Stay hydrated by drinking plenty of water throughout the day. Dehydration can lead to fatigue and decreased energy levels, so it's important to prioritize hydration for optimal well-being.

10. Cultivate Mindfulness and Self-Compassion:

Self-Care Practices: Engage in regular self-care practices that nurture your body, mind, and spirit. Set aside time for activities that bring you joy, relaxation, and fulfillment.

Mindful Awareness: Practice mindfulness by bringing awareness to your thoughts, emotions, and bodily sensations without judgment. Cultivate self-compassion and treat yourself with kindness and understanding.

By implementing these strategies and creating a supportive environment for energy renewal, you can enhance your resilience, boost your vitality, and optimize your overall well-being. Remember to listen to your body's cues, prioritize self-care, and make adjustments as needed to maintain balance and vitality in your life.

Staying Committed to Your Energy Recharge Journey

Staying committed to your energy recharge journey is crucial for maintaining vitality, resilience, and overall well-being. Here are some strategies to help you stay dedicated to your efforts:

1. Set Clear Goals:

Define Your Objectives: Clearly outline your goals and intentions for your energy recharge journey. Identify what you hope to achieve and why it's important to you.

SMART Goals: Make your goals Specific, Measurable, Achievable, Relevant, and Time-bound to provide clarity and motivation for your journey.

2. Create a Sustainable Routine:

Consistent Schedule: Establish a daily or weekly routine that includes regular self-care practices, relaxation techniques, and activities that replenish your energy.

Balance and Variety: Incorporate a variety of activities into your routine to address different aspects of your well-being. Balance restful activities with those that invigorate and energize you.

3. Practice Self-Compassion:

Be Kind to Yourself: Treat yourself with kindness and understanding, especially during challenging times. Acknowledge your efforts and progress, even if you experience setbacks.

Embrace Imperfection: Accept that progress may not always be linear, and that setbacks are a natural part of the journey. Approach yourself with patience and resilience.

4. Stay Flexible and Adaptive:

Adapt to Changes: Remain open to adjusting your approach as needed based on changing circumstances, priorities, and feedback. Flexibility is key to maintaining long-term commitment.

Learn from Challenges: View obstacles and setbacks as opportunities for growth and learning. Use adversity as a chance to develop resilience and refine your strategies.

5. Cultivate Motivation:

Identify Your Why: Connect with your underlying motivations for embarking on your energy recharge journey. Reflect on the benefits and rewards that energizing activities bring to your life.

Visualize Success: Visualize yourself achieving your goals and experiencing the positive outcomes of your efforts. Use visualization techniques to reinforce your commitment and motivation.

6. Seek Accountability and Support:

Share Your Goals: Share your energy recharge goals with trusted friends, family members, or mentors who can offer support, encouragement, and accountability.

Join a Community: Seek out communities or groups of like-minded individuals who share similar goals and values. Engage in discussions, share experiences, and draw inspiration from others.

7. Celebrate Progress:

Acknowledge Achievements: Celebrate your successes, milestones, and progress along the way. Recognize and reward yourself for your commitment and dedication.

Track Your Progress: Keep track of your achievements and milestones to monitor your progress and stay motivated. Celebrate both big and small wins along the journey.

8. Practice Patience and Persistence:

Stay the Course: Remain patient and persistent, even when progress feels slow or challenging. Trust in the process and stay committed to your long-term goals.

Focus on Effort: Shift your focus from immediate results to the effort and dedication you're putting into your energy recharge journey. Trust that consistent effort will yield positive outcomes over time.

9. Reflect and Reassess:

Regular Reflection: Take time to reflect on your journey, assess your progress, and identify areas for improvement. Reflective practice helps you stay aligned with your goals and values.

Adjust Your Approach: Be willing to adjust your strategies and priorities based on your reflections and insights. Continuously refine your approach to better support your energy renewal needs.

10. Stay Inspired:

Find Inspiration: Seek out sources of inspiration that resonate with your values and aspirations. Surround yourself with uplifting stories, quotes, and role models that fuel your motivation.

Reconnect with Purpose: Reconnect with your sense of purpose and passion for your energy recharge journey. Remind yourself of the profound impact that prioritizing self-care and well-being can have on your life.

By integrating these strategies into your energy recharge journey, you can maintain commitment, resilience, and enthusiasm for prioritizing your well-being. Remember that self-care is an ongoing process, and staying dedicated to your energy renewal journey is a powerful investment in your health, happiness, and vitality.

CHAPTER SEVEN

Overcoming Obstacles and Staying on Track

Strategies for Overcoming Setbacks and Challenges

Overcoming setbacks and challenges can be tough, but it's definitely possible with the right strategies. Here are some approaches you can take:

Maintain a Positive Mindset: Cultivate optimism and resilience. Remember that setbacks are a part of life and can provide valuable lessons and opportunities for growth.

Set Realistic Goals: Break down your larger goals into smaller, achievable steps. This can make challenges seem more manageable and help you maintain motivation.

Seek Support: Don't be afraid to lean on friends, family, mentors, or support groups for encouragement and advice during difficult times. Having a support network can make challenges feel less daunting.

Learn from Setbacks: Instead of dwelling on failures, try to analyze what went wrong and what you can learn from the experience. Use setbacks as opportunities for self-reflection and improvement.

Adaptability: Be flexible and open to changing your approach if necessary. Sometimes setbacks occur because our initial plans weren't the best fit for the situation.

Stay Organized and Prioritize: When facing multiple challenges, it can be helpful to organize your tasks and prioritize them based on urgency and importance. This can prevent you from feeling overwhelmed.

Take Care of Yourself: Remember to prioritize self-care, including getting enough sleep, eating healthily, exercising, and managing stress. Taking care of your physical and mental well-being can give you the strength and resilience needed to overcome challenges.

Celebrate Progress: Acknowledge and celebrate even small victories along the way. Recognizing your progress can boost your confidence and motivation to keep moving forward.

Visualize Success: Use visualization techniques to imagine yourself overcoming challenges and achieving your goals. Visualizing success can help you stay focused and motivated during difficult times.

Stay Persistent: Keep pushing forward, even when things get tough. Persistence is key to overcoming setbacks and achieving long-term success.

Remember, setbacks and challenges are inevitable, but how you respond to them ultimately determines your success. By adopting these strategies and maintaining a positive attitude, you can overcome obstacles and emerge stronger than ever.

Cultivating Resilience in the Face of Adversity

Cultivating resilience is essential for navigating through adversity effectively. Here's how you can develop and strengthen your resilience:

Develop a Growth Mindset: Embrace challenges as opportunities for growth rather than viewing them as insurmountable obstacles. Believe in your ability to learn and adapt in the face of adversity.

Practice Self-Compassion: Treat yourself with kindness and understanding, especially during tough times. Accept that it's normal to struggle and make mistakes, and remind yourself that you're doing the best you can.

Build a Strong Support Network: Surround yourself with supportive friends, family members, mentors, and colleagues who can provide encouragement, guidance, and perspective during difficult times. Don't hesitate to reach out for help when you need it.

Develop Problem-Solving Skills: Break down challenges into smaller, more manageable tasks, and approach them systematically. Focus on finding practical solutions rather than getting overwhelmed by the enormity of the problem.

Cultivate Adaptability: Be flexible and willing to adjust your plans and strategies as needed in response to changing circumstances. Adaptability allows you to navigate through uncertainty and bounce back from setbacks more effectively.

Practice Mindfulness and Stress Management: Engage in mindfulness practices such as meditation, deep breathing, or yoga to help calm your mind and reduce stress. Developing self-awareness can also help you better understand your thoughts and emotions in challenging situations.

Maintain a Positive Outlook: Look for the silver lining in difficult situations and focus on what you can control rather than dwelling on things beyond your control. Cultivate gratitude and optimism to help you maintain a positive attitude even during tough times.

Set Realistic Goals: Break down your long-term goals into smaller, achievable steps, and celebrate your progress along the way. Setting realistic goals can help you stay motivated and focused, even when faced with obstacles.

Seek Meaning and Purpose: Reflect on your values, passions, and sense of purpose, and use them as guiding principles to navigate through adversity. Finding meaning in difficult experiences can help you cope with challenges more effectively.

Learn from Adversity: Take time to reflect on your experiences and extract valuable lessons from adversity. Use setbacks as opportunities for personal and professional growth, and apply what you've learned to future challenges.

By incorporating these strategies into your life, you can cultivate resilience and develop the inner strength needed to thrive in the face of adversity. Remember that resilience is a skill that can be developed over time with practice and perseverance.

Maintaining Momentum and Motivation for Lifelong Energy Recharge

Maintaining momentum and motivation for lifelong energy recharge is crucial for sustained success and well-being. Here are some strategies to help you stay energized and motivated:

Set Meaningful Goals: Define clear, compelling goals that align with your values and aspirations. Having a sense of purpose can fuel your motivation and drive.

Break Goals into Manageable Tasks: Break down your goals into smaller, achievable tasks. This makes them less overwhelming and allows you to maintain momentum by focusing on one step at a time.

Create a Routine: Establishing a consistent daily routine can provide structure and help you stay on track. Include activities that energize you, such as exercise, mindfulness practices, and hobbies, to recharge your batteries.

Celebrate Small Wins: Acknowledge and celebrate your progress, no matter how small. Recognizing your achievements boosts morale and reinforces positive habits.

Stay Inspired: Surround yourself with sources of inspiration, whether it's books, podcasts, mentors, or role models. Seek out stories of resilience and success to fuel your motivation during challenging times.

Practice Self-Care: Prioritize self-care activities that nourish your body, mind, and spirit. Get enough sleep, eat healthily, exercise regularly, and make time for relaxation and leisure activities.

Manage Stress: Identify sources of stress in your life and develop healthy coping mechanisms to manage them effectively. This could include techniques such as deep breathing, meditation, or spending time in nature.

Stay Connected: Cultivate supportive relationships with friends, family, and colleagues. Surrounding yourself with positive, like-minded individuals can provide encouragement and motivation when you need it most.

Embrace Continuous Learning: Stay curious and open-minded, and commit to lifelong learning and personal growth. Engage in activities that challenge you intellectually and expand your skills and knowledge.

Reflect and Refocus: Regularly reflect on your progress and reassess your goals to ensure they remain meaningful and relevant. Adjust your strategies as needed and stay flexible in response to changing circumstances.

By incorporating these strategies into your life, you can maintain momentum and motivation for lifelong energy recharge. Remember that it's normal to experience fluctuations in motivation, but with perseverance and dedication, you can stay focused on your goals and continue to thrive.

CHAPTER EIGHT

The Enervate Effect in Action

Real-Life Stories of Transformation and Renewal

Real-life stories of transformation and renewal are powerful reminders of the human capacity for resilience and growth. Here are a few inspiring examples:

J.K. Rowling: Before becoming one of the world's most beloved authors, J.K. Rowling faced numerous setbacks, including joblessness, divorce, and depression. She wrote the first Harry Potter book while struggling as a single mother living on welfare. Despite facing rejection from multiple publishers, Rowling persevered, eventually finding success and transforming her life from hardship to triumph.

Nick Vujicic: Born without arms or legs, Nick Vujicic faced immense physical and emotional challenges growing up. However, he refused to let his disability define him and instead became a motivational speaker, author, and advocate for people with disabilities. Through his message of hope and resilience, Vujicic has inspired millions worldwide to embrace their differences and live life to the fullest.

Malala Yousafzai: Malala Yousafzai defied the Taliban's oppressive regime in Pakistan by advocating for girls' education. In 2012, she survived an assassination attempt at the age of 15 and continued her activism with even greater determination. Malala's courage and resilience led to her becoming the youngest-ever Nobel Peace Prize laureate, and she continues to fight for educational equality and empowerment for girls globally.

Nelson Mandela: Nelson Mandela spent 27 years in prison for his anti-apartheid activism in South Africa. Despite enduring harsh conditions and separation from his family, Mandela remained steadfast in his commitment to justice and reconciliation. Upon his release, he played a pivotal role in ending apartheid and became the country's first democratically elected president, embodying the power of forgiveness and resilience.

Oprah Winfrey: Oprah Winfrey overcame a tumultuous childhood marked by poverty, abuse, and hardship to become one of the most influential media moguls in the world. Through her talk show, philanthropy, and advocacy work, Winfrey has empowered millions to overcome adversity, find their voice, and pursue their dreams.

Steve Jobs: Co-founder of Apple Inc., Steve Jobs was fired from the company he helped build in 1985. However, he didn't let this setback define him. Instead, he went on to found NeXT and Pixar Animation Studios, revolutionizing the computer and entertainment industries. Jobs later returned to Apple, leading it to become one of the most valuable and innovative companies in the world.

Mae Jemison: Mae Jemison shattered barriers as the first African American woman to travel to space. Despite facing racial and gender discrimination throughout her career, she pursued her passion for science and space exploration. Jemison's journey from a small town in Alabama to the stars serves as an inspiration to aspiring scientists and women of color around the world.

Chris Gardner: Chris Gardner's life story was portrayed in the film "The Pursuit of Happyness." After experiencing homelessness and financial hardship while raising his young son, Gardner persevered through countless challenges to become a successful stockbroker and entrepreneur. His resilience and determination to create a better life for himself and his family exemplify the transformative power of perseverance and grit.

Bethany Hamilton: Professional surfer Bethany Hamilton's life changed forever when she lost her left arm in a shark attack at the age of 13. Despite this devastating setback, Hamilton refused to give up her passion for surfing. Through sheer determination and perseverance, she returned to the sport just a month after the attack and went on to become one of the world's top-ranked female surfers. Hamilton's story of resilience and courage has inspired millions to overcome adversity and pursue their dreams.

Jim Carrey: Before achieving fame and success as a comedian and actor, Jim Carrey faced numerous challenges, including financial hardship and his father's unemployment. Carrey used humor as a coping mechanism and pursued his dream of becoming a comedian despite facing rejection and setbacks early in his career. Through his talent, perseverance, and unwavering belief in himself, Carrey rose to become one of Hollywood's most beloved and successful entertainers.

Bethany Hamilton: Professional surfer Bethany Hamilton's life changed forever when she lost her left arm in a shark attack at the age of 13. Despite this devastating setback, Hamilton refused to give up her passion for surfing. Through sheer determination and perseverance, she returned to the sport just a month after the attack and went on to become one of the world's top-ranked female surfers. Hamilton's story of resilience and courage has inspired millions to overcome adversity and pursue their dreams.

Nadia Comăneci: Nadia Comăneci, a Romanian gymnast, made history at the 1976 Olympics when she became the first gymnast to score a perfect 10.0. Despite facing intense pressure and scrutiny, Comăneci remained focused and disciplined, pushing herself to achieve greatness. Her remarkable performance inspired generations of athletes and demonstrated the power of dedication and perseverance in the face of adversity.

Rosa Parks: Often referred to as the "mother of the civil rights movement," Rosa Parks became an icon of resistance and equality when she refused to give up her seat to a white passenger on a segregated bus in Montgomery, Alabama, in 1955. Parks' act of defiance sparked the Montgomery Bus Boycott and galvanized the civil rights movement. Her courage and determination paved the way for significant social and political change, illustrating the transformative impact of standing up for what is right.

J.K. Rowling: Before becoming one of the world's most beloved authors, J.K. Rowling faced numerous setbacks, including joblessness, divorce, and depression. She wrote the first Harry Potter book while struggling as a single mother living on welfare. Despite facing rejection from multiple publishers, Rowling persevered, eventually finding success and transforming her life from hardship to triumph.

Michael Jordan: Widely regarded as one of the greatest basketball players of all time, Michael Jordan faced numerous setbacks and challenges throughout his career. Despite being cut from his high school basketball team, Jordan used rejection as motivation to work harder and prove himself. Through his relentless work ethic, determination, and resilience, Jordan went on to win six NBA championships and earn numerous accolades, inspiring millions around the world to strive for excellence and never give up on their dreams.

Arunima Sinha: Arunima Sinha is the first female amputee to climb Mount Everest. In 2011, she lost her left leg in a tragic accident when she was thrown off a moving train while resisting a robbery attempt. Despite this devastating setback, Sinha refused to be defeated. She underwent multiple surgeries and rehabilitation and trained rigorously to pursue her dream of climbing the world's highest peak. In 2013, she successfully summited Mount Everest, showcasing extraordinary resilience, determination, and courage.

Milkha Singh: Known as the "Flying Sikh," Milkha Singh overcame immense adversity and hardship to become one of India's greatest athletes. Born into poverty and orphaned during the partition of India, Singh faced numerous challenges growing up. However, he found solace in running and went on to represent India in track and field at the Olympics. Singh's remarkable journey from refugee camps to the Olympic arena serves as a testament to the power of perseverance, hard work, and self-belief.

A.P.J. Abdul Kalam: A.P.J. Abdul Kalam, also known as the "Missile Man of India," rose from humble beginnings to become one of the country's most revered scientists and statesmen. Despite facing financial hardships during his childhood, Kalam pursued his passion for aerospace engineering and made significant contributions to India's missile and space programs. He served as the President of India from 2002 to 2007, inspiring millions with his vision, humility, and dedication to serving the nation.

Laxmi Agarwal: Laxmi Agarwal is an Indian acid attack survivor and activist who has become a leading voice in the fight against acid violence and for the rights of survivors. At the age of 15, Agarwal was attacked with acid by a man whose advances she had rejected. Despite enduring physical and emotional trauma, Agarwal refused to hide her face and instead became an advocate for change. She has since campaigned for stricter laws against acid attacks and raised awareness about the issue through public speaking and activism, inspiring countless others to speak out against violence and discrimination.

Sudha Chandran: Sudha Chandran is an accomplished Indian actress and classical dancer who overcame a tragic accident to achieve success in the entertainment industry. At the age of 16, Chandran lost her leg in a car accident. Despite this setback, she continued to pursue her passion for dance, mastering the art of Bharatanatyam with a prosthetic leg. Chandran's determination and resilience propelled her to stardom, and she has since become a role model for people with disabilities, proving that physical limitations are no barrier to achieving one's dreams.

Arunachalam Muruganantham: Arunachalam Muruganantham, also known as the "Padman of India," revolutionized menstrual hygiene in rural India. Concerned about the unaffordable and unhygienic sanitary pads available to women in his village, Muruganantham embarked on a mission to create low-cost sanitary napkins. Despite facing ridicule and ostracization from his community, he persisted in his efforts and eventually developed a simple machine to manufacture affordable pads. His innovation has since improved menstrual health and empowered countless women across India.

Sundar Pichai: Sundar Pichai is the CEO of Alphabet Inc., the parent company of Google. Born and raised in a middle-class family in Chennai, India, Pichai excelled academically and earned a scholarship to attend Stanford

University. He joined Google in 2004 and rose through the ranks to become CEO in 2015. Pichai's journey from a modest upbringing in India to leading one of the world's most influential technology companies serves as a testament to the power of hard work, perseverance, and ambition.

Mary Kom: Mary Kom is an Indian boxer and the only woman to win six World Amateur Boxing Championships. Hailing from a remote village in Manipur, Kom faced numerous obstacles in pursuing her passion for boxing, including financial constraints and societal norms. Despite these challenges, she persisted in her training and went on to achieve remarkable success in the sport. Kom's inspiring journey from a small-town girl to an international boxing icon has inspired millions of aspiring athletes, especially women, across India.

Dr. Prakash Amte and Dr. Mandakini Amte: Dr. Prakash Amte and Dr. Mandakini Amte are Indian social activists and doctors who have dedicated their lives to serving tribal communities in the remote forests of Maharashtra. Despite coming from privileged backgrounds, the couple chose to live and work among the Madia Gond tribe, providing healthcare, education, and social services to marginalized communities. Through their selfless dedication and tireless efforts, they have transformed the lives of thousands of people and inspired others to contribute to social change.

Kailash Satyarthi: Kailash Satyarthi is an Indian children's rights activist who has spent decades fighting against child labor and trafficking. Through his organization, Bachpan Bachao Andolan (Save the Childhood Movement), Satyarthi has rescued thousands of children from bonded labor and exploitation and advocated for their rights on a global scale. His unwavering commitment to protecting the rights and dignity of children has earned him international recognition, including the Nobel Peace Prize in 2014.

Ravi Gulati: Ravi Gulati, also known as the "Water Man of India," dedicated his life to water conservation and rainwater harvesting. Growing up in Rajasthan, Gulati witnessed the devastating effects of water scarcity on rural communities. Determined to make a difference, he founded the NGO Manthan Jan Sewa Sansthan and pioneered innovative techniques for rainwater harvesting and groundwater recharge. Through his efforts, Gulati has transformed arid landscapes into fertile farmland, providing sustainable water solutions to thousands of villages across India.

Sushmita Sen: Sushmita Sen made history in 1994 when she became the first Indian woman to win the Miss Universe pageant. Despite facing skepticism and criticism from society, Sen broke stereotypes and pursued a successful career in Bollywood. Beyond her achievements in the entertainment industry, Sen is known for her philanthropic work and advocacy for women's empowerment and child welfare. Through her foundation, I Am Foundation, she has supported numerous charitable initiatives and inspired others to give back to society.

Dr. Tessy Thomas: Dr. Tessy Thomas, often referred to as the "Missile Woman of India," is a renowned scientist and aerospace engineer. Despite facing gender discrimination in a male-dominated field, Dr. Thomas pursued her passion for rocket technology and played a key role in the development of India's ballistic missile defense program. Her groundbreaking contributions to missile technology have earned her accolades and recognition as a pioneer in the field of aerospace engineering.

Prakash Baskar: Prakash Baskar, also known as the "Solar Man of India," is a social entrepreneur and environmental activist. Concerned about the impact of climate change on rural communities, Baskar founded the NGO GRAAMATHU, which promotes sustainable development through the use of solar energy and eco-friendly technologies. Through his efforts, Baskar has empowered rural households to adopt clean energy solutions, reducing their dependence on fossil fuels and improving their quality of life.

Deepa Malik: Deepa Malik is an Indian athlete and Paralympic medalist who defied the odds to achieve success in sports. Despite being diagnosed with a spinal tumor at the age of 30, Malik refused to let her disability hold her back. She took up para-athletics and went on to win several medals, including a silver medal at the 2016 Paralympic Games in Rio de Janeiro. Malik's resilience and determination have inspired countless individuals with disabilities to pursue their dreams and overcome obstacles.

These stories illustrate the transformative power of resilience, perseverance, and determination in overcoming adversity and achieving personal growth. They serve as reminders that no matter the challenges we face, it is possible to emerge stronger, wiser, and more empowered than before.

Applying the Principles of Energy Recharge to Various Areas of Life

Applying the principles of energy recharge to various areas of life can help you maintain balance, vitality, and fulfillment. Here's how you can incorporate these principles into different aspects of your life:

Physical Health:

Exercise Regularly: Engage in physical activities that you enjoy, such as walking, jogging, yoga, or dancing, to boost your energy levels and promote overall well-being.

Eat Nutritious Foods: Fuel your body with a balanced diet rich in fruits, vegetables, whole grains, lean proteins, and healthy fats to nourish your body and sustain your energy throughout the day.

Prioritize Sleep: Aim for 7-9 hours of quality sleep each night to recharge your body and mind, enhance your mood, and improve cognitive function.

Mental and Emotional Well-being:

Practice Mindfulness: Incorporate mindfulness meditation or deep breathing exercises into your daily routine to reduce stress, increase self-awareness, and cultivate inner peace.

Set Boundaries: Establish clear boundaries in your personal and professional life to protect your time, energy, and mental health from excessive demands and obligations.

Express Gratitude: Take time each day to acknowledge and appreciate the positive aspects of your life, fostering a sense of gratitude that can enhance your overall well-being and resilience.

Career and Professional Development:

Set Realistic Goals: Define clear, achievable goals that align with your values and aspirations, allowing you to focus your efforts and maintain motivation.

Pursue Continuous Learning: Invest in your professional development by acquiring new skills, attending workshops or seminars, and seeking opportunities for growth and advancement.

Seek Work-Life Balance: Strive to maintain a healthy balance between your career and personal life, allocating time for relaxation, hobbies, and meaningful relationships to prevent burnout and sustain your energy over the long term.

Relationships and Social Connections:

Nurture Supportive Relationships: Cultivate strong, supportive connections with family, friends, and colleagues who uplift and inspire you, fostering a sense of belonging and emotional well-being.

Practice Active Listening: Engage in meaningful conversations with others by listening attentively, showing empathy, and offering support, strengthening your relationships and enhancing your social connections.

Schedule Quality Time: Prioritize spending quality time with loved ones, whether it's sharing meals, engaging in recreational activities, or simply enjoying each other's company, to deepen your bonds and recharge your emotional batteries.

Personal Growth and Fulfillment:

Reflect and Self-Assess: Set aside time for self-reflection and introspection to assess your values, goals, and priorities, enabling you to align your actions with your authentic self and cultivate a sense of purpose and fulfillment.

Embrace Creativity: Explore creative outlets such as writing, painting, or music to express yourself, unleash your imagination, and tap into your inner creativity, fostering personal growth and self-expression.

Step Outside Your Comfort Zone: Challenge yourself to try new experiences, take calculated risks, and embrace uncertainty, expanding your horizons and unlocking new opportunities for growth and self-discovery.

By applying the principles of energy recharge to these various areas of your life, you can cultivate a holistic approach to well-being, fulfillment, and resilience, enabling you to thrive and flourish in all aspects of your life.

Inspiring Examples of Living Fully Charged in a Fast-Paced World

Living fully charged in a fast-paced world requires intentionality, balance, and a commitment to well-being. Here are some inspiring examples of individuals who embody this philosophy:

Elon Musk: Elon Musk is known for his relentless drive and ambition as the CEO of SpaceX, Tesla, and other groundbreaking companies. Despite the demanding nature of his work, Musk prioritizes self-care by maintaining a rigorous exercise routine, getting enough sleep, and spending quality time with his family. He emphasizes the importance of maintaining a healthy work-life balance while pursuing ambitious goals.

Arianna Huffington: Arianna Huffington, the co-founder of The Huffington Post, is a vocal advocate for well-being and mindfulness in the workplace. After experiencing burnout firsthand, Huffington transformed her approach to life and work, prioritizing sleep, meditation, and self-care. She founded Thrive Global, a company dedicated to helping individuals and organizations prioritize well-being and performance in a fast-paced world.

Richard Branson: Richard Branson, the founder of the Virgin Group, leads a dynamic and adventurous lifestyle while maintaining a strong focus on well-being and balance. He emphasizes the importance of staying active, spending time outdoors, and fostering meaningful connections with others. Branson believes that living a fulfilling life involves pursuing passions, taking calculated risks, and prioritizing personal happiness.

Sheryl Sandberg: Sheryl Sandberg, the COO of Facebook, is a prominent advocate for work-life balance and resilience. Following the sudden death of her husband, Sandberg became a vocal proponent of building resilience in the face of adversity. She emphasizes the importance of leaning on support networks, practicing self-compassion, and finding meaning in difficult circumstances. Sandberg's openness about her personal struggles has inspired others to prioritize well-being and resilience in their own lives.

Tim Ferriss: Tim Ferriss, author of "The 4-Hour Workweek" and host of "The Tim Ferriss Show" podcast, is known for his unconventional approach to productivity and lifestyle design. Ferriss advocates for optimizing work and leisure activities to maximize efficiency and fulfillment. He emphasizes the importance of setting boundaries, practicing mindfulness, and focusing on activities that bring joy and meaning.

These individuals demonstrate that it is possible to thrive in a fast-paced world while prioritizing well-being, balance, and fulfillment. By embracing a holistic approach to life and work, they inspire others to live fully charged and pursue their passions with purpose and intentionality.

Epilogue

In the final chapter of "The Enervate Effect: Recharging Your Life's Battery," we conclude our journey of exploration into the transformative power of energy renewal. As we reflect on the principles, practices, and stories shared throughout this book, we are reminded of the profound impact that prioritizing self-care and rejuvenation can have on our lives.

In this epilogue, we take a moment to celebrate the progress made and the lessons learned on our path toward greater vitality and well-being. We acknowledge the challenges overcome, the habits cultivated, and the resilience built along the way.

We also recognize that the journey toward sustained energy is not without its setbacks and obstacles. Life's demands and unforeseen circumstances may test our commitment to self-care, but we are equipped with the tools and knowledge to navigate these challenges with grace and determination.

As we bid farewell to these pages, we are filled with a sense of hope and possibility for the future. Armed with a deeper understanding of our own energy needs and the importance of balance in our lives, we step forward with confidence and intentionality.

May this book serve as a guiding light on your continued journey toward vitality and fulfillment. May you always remember the power of the Enervate Effect and the transformative impact it can have on every aspect of your life.

With heartfelt gratitude and best wishes for your ongoing success.

.....***.....